Art Therapy, Dreams, and Healing: Beyond the Looking Glass

Art Therapy, Dreams, and Healing: Beyond the Looking Glass synthesises methods to work with one's dreams through art therapy and introduces the reader to brief creative methods, Gestalt and Jungian experiential methods, and research on lucid dreaming and dream re-entry.

The author provides a unique, clear and concise synthesis of 19 available dreamwork methods to find the message of your dreams, with examples from her own 35 years of psychotherapy practice. Along with a classification of types and functions of dreams, chapters include information such as how to keep a dream journal, how to remember one's dreams, how to identify 25 different dream types and how to follow your own dreamwork process.

This book provides a succinct blend of available dreamwork methods for readers to find the existential message of their dreams and grow from them.

Johanne Hamel is a psychologist and art psychotherapist who has been teaching art therapy for 20 years in university programs in Canada. She is currently an international lecturer in Thailand, the USA and Europe. More information can be found at her website johannehamel.com.

Hélène Hamel is a self-employed translator who holds an Honors degree in translation and has been working mainly from English to French for more than 30 years. She occasionally accepts translation work from French to English. Over the years, she has developed a great interest in therapy practices and alternative medicine, and the publishing world is where she is now heading. She can be reached at hamhel444@outlook.com.

W0113677

"Readers interested in dreaming and dream interpretation need a good book on using art therapy and time-honored techniques for dreamwork, and Johanne Hamel has the qualifications, experience and skills to make that a reality!"

Robert Waggoner, author of *Lucid Dreaming – Gateway to the Inner Self* and co-author of *Lucid Dreaming Plain and Simple*

"This book offers a unique, indispensable integration of art therapy, psycho-therapy and dreamwork but is not limited to that; it also encompasses writing methods, lucid dreaming, and other aspects of creativity. As a long-time dream journalist, and a psychologist, I am intrigued by this book very much and I am sure that it would attract and inspire many other readers as well."

Misa Tsuruta, PhD, psychologist/psychotherapist (Tokyo, Japan)

"Already published in French, the success, uniqueness and clear depiction of this book on Art Therapy and Dreams makes it a valuable contribution to the field. Johanne Hamel's many years of experience in the field as a mental health professional has given her the insight and the expertise required to write on this topic. Her many years of involvement in the art therapy field, her books and her research, have spread the knowledge of dream work to many parts of the world including Thailand, where she teaches on a regular basis."

Lucille Proulx, MA, ATR, RCAT, Canadian International Institute of Art Therapy

Art Therapy, Dreams, and Healing

Beyond the Looking Glass

Johanne Hamel

Translated by Hélène Hamel

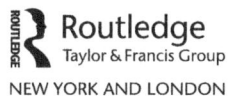

Routledge
Taylor & Francis Group

NEW YORK AND LONDON

Originally published in French as:
Rêves, Art-Thérapie et Guérison, De l'autre côté du miroir
© 2017, Québec Livres, division of Groupe Sogides Inc. (Montréal, Québec, Canada)
All rights reserved

First published 2021
by Routledge
52 Vanderbilt Avenue, New York, NY 10017

and by Routledge
2 Park Square, Milton Park, Abingdon, Oxon, OX14 4RN

Routledge is an imprint of the Taylor & Francis Group, an informa business

© 2021 Taylor & Francis

Library of Congress Cataloging-in-Publication Data
Names: Swan-Foster, Nora, editor.
Title: Art therapy and childbearing issues / edited by Nora Swan-Foster.
Description: New York, NY : Routledge, 2020. | Includes bibliographical references and index. |
Identifiers: LCCN 2020011477 (print) | LCCN 2020011478 (ebook) | ISBN 9780367436513 (hardback) | ISBN 9780367436506 (paperback) | ISBN 9781003004837 (ebook)
Subjects: LCSH: Art therapy. | Mothers--Mental health. | Pregnant women--Mental health. | Mothers--Counseling of. | Pregnant women--Counseling of.
Classification: LCC RC489.A7 A767 2020 (print) | LCC RC489.A7 (ebook) |
DDC 616.89/1656--dc23
LC record available at https://lccn.loc.gov/2020011477
LC ebook record available at https://lccn.loc.gov/2020011478

ISBN: 978-0-367-46045-7 (hbk)
ISBN: 978-0-367-46044-0 (pbk)
ISBN: 978-1-003-02662-4 (ebk)

Typeset in Sabon and Helvetica Neue
by Servis Filmsetting Ltd, Stockport, Cheshire

Dedication

This book is especially dedicated to all my art psychotherapy clients and art therapy students who worked their dreams with me along all these years and thus helped me develop these methods to elucidate their meanings. Thank you to all of you. With love, Johanne Hamel.

Contents

List of Figures

Foreword

Having a dream is natural.
Working with a dream can be ... magical and life changing!

Every night, you spend almost 23% of your sleep time in the realm of dreaming. This means that by the time you are 11 years old, you have spent almost one complete year in the realm of dreams. But what do you understand of dreaming and your personal dream symbolism? Often, very little.

Through dream work techniques, like those in this book by Johanne Hamel D. Ps., you have the opportunity to explore dream imagery firsthand. You will discover that embedded in your dream symbols is something meaningful and significant. By working with your dreams, you will begin to see their extraordinary creativity, insight and energy – and how dreams can serve to illuminate the path to your fullest life.

Although I write books on lucid dreaming (which means realising within the dream that you are dreaming), I routinely encourage people to learn how to work with dream symbols and uncover their meaning. Even in a lucid dream, it helps to understand the language of dream symbolism so you can benefit from your encounters with dream figures and dream objects when lucid.

At a lucid dreaming workshop in Taiwan, a woman asked me, "I seem unable to lose weight, no matter how hard I try. Can lucid dreaming help me lose weight?" I told her that I believed it could. However, she did not need to have a lucid dream to discover how to lose weight. She could simply incubate or request a dream tonight, which would explain to her the underlying reason for her inability to lose weight.

That night, she asked to have a dream which would show her why she could not lose weight.

In the morning, she told the lucid dream workshop participants, "Last night, I asked to have a dream that would explain why I could not lose weight. Then I dreamt that I was a puffer fish – the kind of fish that gets bigger when it feels threatened, so that the other fish will not bother it." Some laughter and smiles appeared among the crowd as people began to 'get' the dream's symbolic message.

The dreamer concluded, "Now I understand why I do not lose weight. My dream has shown me that I hold onto my weight so that others will not push me around. My weight is a defense mechanism." With the help of this dream symbol, she came to a much deeper understanding of something that had bothered her for many years.

The creativity and wisdom of the unconscious is so profound that it can call forth one dream symbol, the puffer fish, to convey the reasoning behind her issue with weight and show it as a natural defense mechanism against being pushed around. With that knowledge of the underlying reason, this woman could now focus on resolving the real issue (and not its exterior expression of holding onto weight).

Dreamwork is like art. It helps to approach it from the heart. To listen to your intuitive voice. To see what comes up in your imagination. And perhaps most importantly to simply play with the dream symbols and the unconscious mind.

In this book, you will find many methods to work, draw *and play* with dream symbols. When you suddenly have that 'aha' moment, then you will know that you are getting it – you are learning from your dreaming self and seeing its wisdom, beauty and creativity.

Best wishes on your journey into dreamwork!

Robert Waggoner
Author of *Lucid Dreaming – Gateway to the Inner Self*
and co-author of *Lucid Dreaming Plain and Simple*

Preface

Art Therapy, Dreams, and Healing

Published for the first time in 1993 and sub-headed « Journal de croissance personnelle par le rêve et l'art » *(Personal Development Journal through dreaming and art)*, this book remains current for the clinical information it provides as well as for the psychotherapeutic importance of dreamwork, which is and will always be a very profound tool for self-knowledge and transformation. Therefore, it was worth updating and editing it in English.

Art Therapy, Dreams, and Healing: Each of these concepts refers to an aspect of my professional practice.

Dreams

Even after 40 years of practice, I witness time and again the effectiveness of this personal and professional tool. This efficiency comes from the transformative power of symbols, which emerge naturally through dreams and artwork. Dreamwork is and will always be an invaluable tool in my art psychotherapy practice.

Art therapy

Drawing or painting a dream has an impact on the patient's psyche and a therapeutic effect that goes beyond words. Combined with dreaming, art therapy is an outstanding healing art since its impact on the patient's psyche is intensified by the visual representation of the dream.

Healing

Using the word "healing" often leaves an uncomfortable feeling. Therefore, it is important to give a definition of this word for the purpose of this book. Jung (1976) defines psychological healing as a process leading to gradually recovering one's integrity as well as forgotten or unconscious parts of oneself. He considers that human beings are born complete and they forget more and more parts of themselves over time as a result of socialisation and fortuitous circumstances. He understands psychological healing as a progressive integration of one's potentials and a harmonisation of one's inner conflicts. One of the therapeutic effects of psychic work is to help us get out of our misery, as Jung (1976) states about art when encouraging his patients to draw images seen in dreams:

"In fact, a singular power originates from the images drawn by a dreamer, and this is not easily described. For example, if a patient noted many times that creating a symbolic image brings a release from a miserable psychic condition, he will turn to it each time he enters into a poor state of mind" (p. 124).[1]

For Jung, symbols and their transformative power are the driving forces of a dream's images, what he refers to as the "transcendent function". For him, symbols have an expressive aspect, which means they express the psychic reality of an individual, and they also have a reactive aspect. The reactive aspect means that an individual reacts to his own expression which is of paramount importance in art therapy.

In its broadest sense, the word *healing* refers to facilitating the individuation process, by which we continuously seek our expression and our accomplishment as the unique individual who lies deep within.

In this book, the word *healing* also refers to a potential physical recovery, in the sense that dreams can address our physical condition and how to heal ourselves. How could it be otherwise given that the body cannot be separated from psyche? Healing one is healing the other. Mrs Patricia Garfield (1991), one of the most prolific and knowledgeable authors about dreamwork, emphasises that healing can turn out to be an emotional and spiritual rebirth, even more so than physical. As she indicates, if you are critically ill or severely injured, you are embarking on an inner healing process and a significant inner journey.

Whether you are ill or healthy, this book is inviting you to a crucial exploration journey and to look *beyond the looking glass.*

Johanne Hamel, January 2020.

---

[1] Free translation.

Acknowledgments

I am very grateful to every person who generously contributed their dream to this book: Brigitte, Carole, Catherine, Claude, Denise, Francine, Gilberte, José, Madeleine, Mario, Pierrette, Sonia ... among others ...

A special thank you to Robert Waggoner who wrote the preface of this book, and to my sister Hélène Hamel who worked very professionally to translate my book from French to English!

Thank you to my husband and to my children, Félix and Catherine, whose constant support and love give the deepest meaning to my life.

Introduction

The Clown In the Mirror

I am walking into a room and I am standing in front of a mirror where I can see a male figure. The man is moving as if trying to see me. Just as I turn my back on him, a dressing mirror appears and I can see this man from his back, apparently walking away. I realise that it is a work of art in two distinct parts and I find the idea interesting. When I look again, the man now appears to be a clown.

Excerpt from a Dialogue Between the Dreamer and the Clown Character

Dreamer: *Mirror, who are you?*

Mirror: *I am a living mirror. Within me, there is a figure moving and coming alive; I am proposing a double reflection to play a trick on you; I am the reflection of your soul.*

Dreamer: *What about you, Mr. Clown, who are you?*

Clown: *I am an image showing up when you are least expecting it; I keep appearing, disappearing and coming back in another mirror; I catch you down the road; I am a fugitive image on the move and I am difficult to capture. I am intangible as I belong to the mirror; you cannot capture me or touch me, but I am here, mysterious and elusive.*

Dreamer: *When I look away from the first mirror, you appear in the second one, pretending you are walking away!*

Clown: *Right! I am leaving when you turn your eyes away from me. But if you look at me again, I am here! And when I am turning my back on you, I am inviting you to follow me. In fact, I am checking if you are following me!*

Dreamer: *What do you want from me?*

Clown: *I am just like you; I am mimicking your gestures. But I am also different; I move and I have a life of my own. Now it's time for you to follow me and to make my gestures. Come with me, I will show you the way. Come and see beyond the looking glass ...*

Dreamer: *Okay, this time I will follow you on this journey into the unknown ... this exciting adventure that is calling me to follow my own destiny.*

Dreamer's comments

In this dream, the clown character represents the Self in the Jungian sense – in other words the sacred part of our being, intangible but ever present if we are willing to make way for it instead of turning our back on it. The Self is the part calling us to our spirituality and to greater fulfillment. This dream shows clearly that the clown is inviting me to follow him at a decisive moment in my life when I was considering leaving my job to start my own private practice.

What the Dream Is ...

However, the clown character might also be interpreted as the dream express-ing itself, because the clown's language gives a clear picture of the dream's reality. Actually, the following words might be the better description of the dream: A fugitive and intangible image, both mysterious and elusive, catching us down the road and reflecting the soul. While having a life of his own, the clown makes our gestures and invites us to follow him, to explore beyond the looking glass, the hidden face of our being ... He vanishes if we turn our back on him, but willingly comes back if we show an interest, as dreams are more easily recalled when we show an interest and take time to jot them down.

This book was inspired by this dream. At first a simple notebook for dreams, it rapidly expanded to elucidate many methods allowing exploration of the dream world.

Nineteen clinical and art-therapy methods for dreamwork are put together in this book. In a sense, the book offers a synthesis of the main techniques used in dreamwork and of the information dispersed across specialised litera-ture on the subject. My focus was to make readily available the methods that supported me and my clients personally and professionally throughout our journey into the dreaming realm. I chose the ones I considered very efficient: Brief approaches, experiential methods or art-therapy methods. For clarity and efficiency purposes, they were simplified as much as possible.

The first edition of this book addressed an important need as books on the subject were not only uncommon, but also generally limited to dream dictionaries. This book's original character lies in its art-therapy approaches, including one based on sounds and movements of the dream. This last new approach was created by Mrs. Michelle Rinfret, a colleague and friend. With regard to approaches based on artwork, few authors gave specific indications as to how dream artwork should be done and about finding an existential message in dreams. But we learned with Sigmund Freud and Carl Jung that drawing a dream's images is possible.

Furthermore, this book's proposed method of keeping a Dream Journal and the indications on how to use the Gestalt dialogue are both original. A dual approach is used in my art-therapy methods as well as in the entire book, as it is inspired by the humanistic/Gestalt and the Jungian, psychodynamic approaches.

While this book is focused on individual dreamwork, working on a dream can nevertheless be hazardous; when embarking on such a journey, it might be wise to seek professional help if needed. If ever you feel troubled or lost, and experience a flood of emotions impeding your functional ability, ask for help from an art therapist, a psychologist or a professional psychotherapist, to help you go through these intense moments of personal growth. However, the individuals going through some transformation are usually able to modulate the rhythm of their journey to avoid sudden or disturbing changes. For personal inner work, do not hesitate to set your own pace.

In the following pages, I am never inviting you to seek to *understand* the meaning of a dream, as it refers to intellectual processes. I rather invite you *to grasp the existential message*, which is a Gestalt concept. Doing this has a broader scope, as *grasping the existential message* means perceiving in your deepest self and beyond any doubt what your dream uncovers about the way you experience human existence. This involves re-entering the dream realm and allowing yourself to be moved by what the dream's images and symbols seek to reveal. This is not an intellectual *puzzle* requiring some kind of decoding with a dream dictionary. In fact, only the dreamer is capable of identifying the existential message carried by his dream, because only the dreamer can assess if the words coming up into his mind reflect clearly his feelings and the images in his dream.

But why should we spend time trying to find the dream's existential message? For those times when something opens up and we discover another part of ourselves, someone familiar and yet unknown, living in a universe both invisible and real! These moments give us a different perception of ourselves and lead us to contemplate a broad range of possibilities unseen before. Knowing who we really are and feeling a connection with ourselves are somehow very gratifying experiences.

What we are looking for through our search for the dream's existential message is a heightened self-awareness. We are all walking next to ourselves, just like zombies, unaware of what is motivating us and affecting us the most. Our inner world is rich with experiences and unexplored potentials; it is unveiling itself through our dreams, through imagination and through art. The approaches proposed in this book offer many gateways to this inner realm.

In this book, I also place great emphasis on lucid dreaming, as a privileged means for consciousness development. Since we dream as we live and since we can learn to live as we dream, training ourselves to become aware of our night dreaming can lead to us demonstrating a greater lucidity when being awake. Charles T. Tart (1986) would say we develop a higher state of consciousness called *genuine self-consciousness* which I personally call *self-presence*. We then become more and more complete, and our rational, our imaginary and our emotional and spiritual worlds become less and less compartmentalised. We also become more complex, fulfilled and creative. Essentially, personal growth truly means using our potential, owning our inner richness and living joyfully.

1

Dreams and Existential Messages

As we start writing down our dreams, we get fascinated by the dream world, this mysterious inner realm rich with images and symbols. Keeping a Dream Journal is one of the best ways of getting to know oneself and realising one's potential.

In this chapter, numerous examples are given to illustrate this point. Using a classification of the different types of dreams, I will give real-life examples, explaining for each type of dream what the dreamer learned about himself. The generally recognised functions of dreams will also be addressed.

Writing Down One's Dreams

The very act of keeping a Dream Journal, which consists of writing down one's dreams day after day, generates major changes in self-consciousness. Sharing one's night dream with a close one in the morning has the same impact. However, writing down one's dreams highlights the similarities in our personal symbols in the long term, therefore understanding their evolution. As a demonstration of this enriching process, here is an excerpt of a Dream Journal kept by a 37-year-old organisational development consultant:

I noticed all kinds of beneficial effects in those times when I was actively keeping my Dream Journal. I noticed a greater self-consciousness and a more acute knowledge of my inner world during the night as well as during the day. During the night, I experienced an occasional lucid dream and during the day, I noticed I was paying closer attention to the fantasy images arising spontaneously in my mind. Consequently, the day and night imaginary worlds were no longer so separated. And as a result, my waking life became substantially enriched, as if a door had opened onto a wonderful world. I also got increasingly aware that there was more to me than my usual logical and rational self, in other words the self required for adaptation to the physical and social environment.

That is to say, the very act of writing down one's dreams is a great learning experience. However, keeping a Dream Journal should be fun and never become a constraint. After a while, you will get into your own rhythm in regard to writing down your dreams and doing dreamwork. Each individual has his/her own pace which also varies with how busy he/she is in their personal and professional life. There are times when it is just impossible to attend to one's dreams.

Personally, I usually write down eight dreams each month, which is a small number, and I work on half of them, which is a lot for me. I do not spend all day working on my dreams, but considering they provide a lot of information about my inner life, I use them consistently for personal transformation. This pace is suited to me and my lifestyle. At other times, when I am particularly in need of understanding what I am going through, I can write down thirty or forty dreams per month. It is up to you to find your own suitable rhythm. To use this self-growth tool successfully, there is no need to spend a tremendous amount of time taking note of each and every one of your dreams.

The Existential Message, Potential for Self-Growth …

In addition to jotting down your dreams, dreamwork can obviously help in understanding the existential message they carry. Dreams tell you about your personal dynamics and the matters going on inside of you which ultimately impact all the important decision making in your life and your significant relationships. This principle generally applies to any dream, although different types of dreams may have slightly different functions.

Dream Types and Their Functions

The classification of dreams proposed here is based on what is commonly offered in the specialised literature. A brief definition is given for each dream type and its generally recognised function, followed by an example and the existential message associated with it.

Symbolic Dreams

This is the most common dream type. It is filled with weird or inconsistent imagery and its successive events do not seem to have any common thread. The message has a symbolic form and its symbols need to be decoded. Carl Jung (1993, 1974), a famous Swiss psychiatrist and one of Freud's colleagues, specifies that this type of dreams can have many functions:

- A **self-regulating** function. The dream is rectifying a situation, adding what the situation is missing or what was repressed or neglected in conscious life experiences, during waking life;

- A **compensatory** function for conscious attitudes. The dream illustrates a perspective or a situation utterly opposite to a conscious experience, which is called by Jung an "extreme conscious attitude". The dream seeks to restore a balance;
- A **compensatory** function for repressed desires. While it is now generally recognised that Freud largely exaggerated the importance of repressed sexual desire, the fact is that some dreams have an effective compensatory effect for sexual desire or for all kinds of different desires not clearly perceived in waking life;
- A **support** function for conscious activity (a function considered as quite uncommon according to Jung). The dream reinforces a direction the dreamer wants to take in waking life. He does not gain new information from dreamwork, but gains confidence in the decision he is about to take;
- A **prospective** function. The dream is an anticipation of future conscious activity. Jung observed this phenomenon in the early stages of some of his clients' psychotherapy process. He called this the *initial dream*; the dream has a prognostic value, which means it is offering invaluable information about the direction and probable results of the therapy process.

Symbolic dreams, clear dreams and hypnagogic dreams usually seek to draw attention to one aspect of our past experience that went unnoticed. As for other dream types addressed further, additional functions are associated with them.

Example of a symbolic dream: A grandmother had the following night dream

Going Back to the Convent

I am with past friends and colleagues in the convent where I studied in my youth. My best friend Estelle is sitting beside me. Our school desks have two seats and their lid can be opened like the ones for young kids. My books are inside the desk, and there are burners to cook food on the desktop. We feel very excited as we can cook anything we want. Being with my friends makes me feel extremely good and it brings back the sense of wellness I had when I was with them in the convent. I am cooking potatoes and I don't care even if they are burning, being sure they will taste good anyways!

Comments

The dreamer had this dream after sharing meals with friends and family on Easter Sunday and Monday. When she recalls these meals, the feeling is the same than in her dream, a sense of well-being when sharing a meal with close ones. In addition, she intends to invite one of her friends to a restaurant in the next few days.

Here, the dream's function is a compensatory one to cope with an unfulfilled desire. The dreamer feels sad because these festive occasions happen much too infrequently to her liking; her dream is a reminder that she is missing the kind of occasions that make her feel so good. Therefore, the dream's existential message is that she finds it important to nurture festive occasions where she can do what she likes doing with friends. Chances are that these moments will make her feel like she is recapturing her youth.

Clear Dreams

Clear dreams are the opposite of symbolic ones. In this case, everything is totally clear, as the dream depicts an event with a factual message. It contains very little weird or incongruous imagery. Its purpose is to draw attention on some aspect of a past situation that went unnoticed. For example, it could be one did not pay attention to a specific emotion experienced during the day. The *literal dream* is another type of clear dream where a dreamer sees himself carrying out day-to-day activities.

Example of a clear dream

Saying "No" to My Father

I am sitting down for a meal with my family of origin. My father is present. I get angry with him and declare that I am now 36 years old and a grown-up adult able to make my own decisions.

Dreamer's comments

No need for decoding this dream. It shows clearly that I am distancing myself from the values attached to my father in order to make my own choices. I had this dream following a clear decision to reduce my workload. I always saw my father as working very hard and attaching a great deal of importance to his career, sometimes at the expense of his own well-being. I was therefore making a different choice. This dream showed I was getting away from learned values to choose new ones more in line with who I now was. It was illuminating an unconscious aspect of me: I was unaware of how much I had been influenced by my father's values and of the impact on my professional decisions. I now had greater control over the factors consciously or unconsciously influencing my career choices. This dream had a self-regulating function by adding a piece of information my conscious self was missing.

Hypnagogic Dreams

Hypnagogic dreams occur in a light stage of sleep or when waking up. Images produced by our imagination just before falling asleep or before waking up are called *hypnagogic* and can be used just the same as for any other dream. This dream type has the same functions as symbolic dreams.

Example of a hypnagogic dream

One day, just before getting out of bed and waking up, the following images went through my mind.

The Native American Blazon

I am seeing a "Native American Blazon" with an oval shape made of deer skin and mounted on a wooden structure. At the center, a pocket looks like a kangaroo pouch. I intuitively know it depicts the "East Blazon".

Dreamer's comments

For my dreamwork on this hypnagogic dream, I designed a three-dimensional piece of art (See Figure 1.1). At that time, I was very inspired by Native

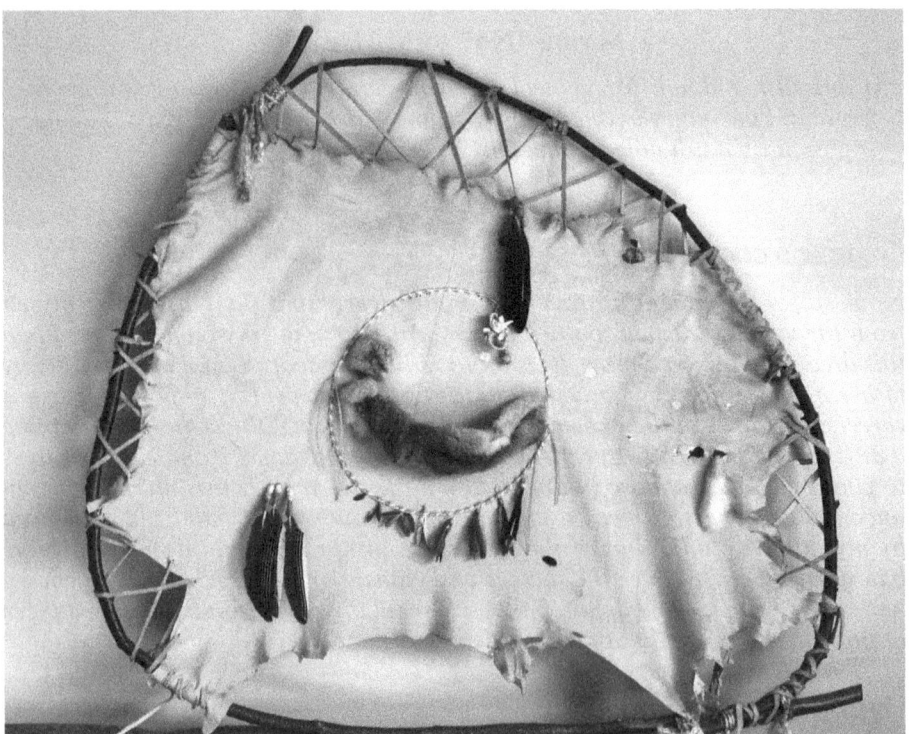

Figure 1.1 *Native American Blazon*. 120 cm × 120 cm (4' × 4'). Tree branches, deer skin, rabbit skin, feathers, fabric, ribbon, wool, beads and crystals.

American spirituality and I knew about the Native American tradition which consists of designing a blazon for each of the four cardinal points, for the purpose of spiritual growth. Blazons speak about who we are and the qualities and personality traits we are offering to the world. It is a symbolic affirmation of one's identity.

This Blazon accompanied me throughout my first pregnancy and afterwards. Every action taken to create this piece of art took on a meaning regarding the profound human experience of giving birth. Every piece of it made sense, from the rabbit skin, a fertility symbol for me, to the umbilical cord that I cut a while after my child was born. Creating this Blazon helped me to understand the meaning of this experience and to overcome my fears and worries concerning motherhood. As it also enabled me to express my experience through symbols, a genuine dialogue was made possible between me and the Blazon.

This hypnagogic dream had a prospective function, as it was telling me in advance of my pregnancy and thus getting me prepared for it. Creating the Blazon played a self-regulating role by helping me to realise over time what I was going through during my pregnancy and after childbirth.

Initial Dreams

As previously indicated, in his book *La guérison psychologique* (1993) (Psychological Healing, 1993), Jung addresses initial dreams, in other words dreams occurring in the early stages of a psychotherapy treatment. He would deliberately pay attention to the first dreams recounted by his patients, because he was convinced that they were containing potential information on their issues or conveying some premonition or indication about their psychological development potential. These dreams might for example reveal forgotten or repressed memories bringing to the surface *virtual possibilities for personality development trapped somewhere in the past*[1] or they might refer to some present conditions existing in the dreamer's life causing problems he is not aware of.

Example of an initial dream

The Five Suitcases

In my dream, I am seeing five big suitcases, each one having a different color and a different size. I am saying to someone that everything is ready.

---

1 Free translation.

Comments

My client had this dream just before her fourth therapy session and we worked on it up to the ninth session of the therapy process. In each new session, she would draw a suitcase with a different color, allowing the symbolic images it contained to spontaneously arise in her mind. Five significant issues came up and were worked on deeply in different ways over the three-and-a-half year span of her therapy process. The words stating "*Everything is ready*" made reference to the dreamer's willingness to work on specific therapeutic issues which were to open up herself to love, to make room for her need for a sense of belonging, to develop her inner strength and to reconnect with her inner child. With the last suitcase came a mandala, a symbol for integration of the psyche. The fact it emerged with the last suitcase was significant, after the dreamer worded the first four issues that she would be working through over the therapy process.

Considering that an initial dream can help identifying issues, solutions and sometimes a positive or negative prognostic within a psychotherapy process, it might be important for the dreamer to elucidate its meaning to have an idea of the forthcoming psychological work. The dream may even inform the dreamer whether the chosen therapist is the right one, as might suggest a negative prognostic. For the psychotherapist, it is also interesting to see at an early stage the issues to be worked on with the patient.

Nightmares

A nightmare is a symbolic dream which can leave highly intense feelings of fear, terror or anxiety upon waking up. Typically, the dreamer is being chased hostilely by a human, an animal figure or a monster, or he feels helpless because of life threatening situations like suffocation, falling down through the air, drowning, paralysis, loss of control, feeling lost or humiliated in public (for example, failing publicly an exam). Nightmares can also be about traumas with images depicting past traumatic experiences, like a car accident, a war scene (for veterans) or any other event about threats of death or injury. Nightmares are very important for our personal growth as they offer an opportunity for working on many traumatic or unconscious aspects.

Example of a nightmare: A 60-year-old person had the following dream

Risk of Flooding

Everybody around me says we need a boat because we are facing a risk of flooding. There is a small boat left behind that nobody is claiming. My partner and I decide to take it over to fill it with all the needed survival equipment. I realise that the boat must have at least four seats so that my

children can come with us. I am thinking of a few articles to take with me, but I have difficulty reasoning because my brain is slow in the face of danger. We need oars for the boat, food, water and canvasses to protect us from the sun. The boat looks operational and heavy. In fact, when I look from closer, I can see it rather looks like a pedal boat without pedals. It is equipped with four seats with two of them being rear facing.

Further ahead, there is a much bigger boat that belongs to one of my sisters. It feels like she has been preparing for the flooding for a long time. On her boat, there are many children as well as one of my nieces and a number of other persons. It looks much more efficient than ours. At one point, my sister falls in the water and drowns. I realise that there will be a lot of orphans.

I woke up crying following this dream predicting the end of the world, realising I would need a boat to come out alive of the flooding.

Comments

After working on this, the dreamer came up with the conclusion she had to let go of something coming to an end in her life, despite her sadness and mixed feelings and the impression she was leaving people behind, probably her present job …

Anxiety Dreams

This dream type symbolically illustrates the psychic anxiety the dreamer bears within. It is not as extreme as a nightmare and the dream's intensity does not cause the dreamer to wake up, but he awakes with feelings of discomfort and considerable uneasiness.

Example of an anxiety dream: A young 23-year-old woman had the following recurring dream

The Bridge in a Void

I see a big void with a very sharp and eroded rock at the center. Above the rock, it is very dark and foggy with a gloomy atmosphere. I see a bridge made of wooden planks without pillars and looking suspended within the void, as a way to get there. It is not sturdy as wooden planks are broken and filled with holes. I have to walk across the bridge to get to the sharp rock at the center and I feel afraid to go on. After a few steps, I glance towards the mainland, trying to hold on to the thread edge. I just cannot make up my mind, feeling unable to decide if I want to go on or go back. I wake up with a feeling of uneasiness.

Comments

This young woman was bullied for her slight overweight in primary school and her acne in secondary school. Having heard all kinds of hurtful things about her, she developed a lack of self-confidence and could only envision a gloomy future at that time.

Death Dreams

There are three types of dreams about death: Dreams where we die, where we meet death itself and where we meet a deceased person. These are different from grieving dreams allowing to deal with our feelings and to go through the grieving process about a deceased loved one.

Dreams Where We Die

A dream where we die is often distressing. The dreamer is wondering if it announces his own death. Jung (2010) affirms there is nothing dangerous about these dreams. Experience taught me they rather indicate the end of a life cycle, a time of transition or the need to let go of something.

Dreams Announcing Death

As for dreams really announcing death, they are of a different kind. A friend of mine who had cancer and knew she was dying had the following dream. If you have such a dream, please remember any dream must always be interpreted within one's own context! Please refrain from concluding right away that it is predicting your own death.

Example of a dream announcing death

The Black Candles

In my dream, I see a series of burning black candles and it smells of putrefaction.

Meeting Death Itself

Dreams where death itself is personified must be interpreted taking into account the specific context. For example, a dreamer met a death figure two times, the first encounter occurring after learning his partner had cancer. Following these two dreams, he assumed his partner would probably die or there was little hope for her healing. As a matter of fact, she passed away a few years later, as the result of generalised cancer.

Examples of two dreams meeting death

Death Knocks at My Door

I am lying on my left side on the inside doormat at home. It is a dark night and there are no lights in the house. Through the side windows, I see a starry sky. Stars are so bright that the floor besides me is illuminated by a strip of light. I realise I cannot move as my arms and my legs are so heavy it feels like my body is paralysed. As I lift my eyes to the door's window, I notice someone is watching me. He is holding still and perfectly straight. Because he is silhouetted against the shining stars, only his face and his eyes are visible, and they are even brighter than the stars; I also notice he is wearing a hat. I am starting to panic, begging him to leave ...

Death Comes My Way

It all starts with a recurring dream. After spending a long time walking, I get to the edge of Quebec City, deep in the countryside. It is winter, everything is covered in snow and I can see cliffs and the river. I am wondering why I got back there once again, while being aware it's a dream. Made of wire mesh, the floor under my feet starts shaking all of a sudden; as I turn around, I realise I am on a ferry boat and already far from shore. In front of me, a man is standing on the deck of the boat and I assume it's the captain. I tell him I am not supposed to be on his ferry, and I want him to turn around and go back to shore. Holding still and showing no reaction at all, the man just keeps looking at me. I start panicking.

I know death itself is looking at me in this dream.

Meeting a Deceased Person

Another type of dream about death is the one where we meet a deceased loved one (see Garfield, 1997), which is very intriguing for dreamers. As these dreams commonly occur following death, it could imply some telepathic communication. They can occur a few weeks or months following death and even years later. Typically, the deceased person is coming in to say goodbye and to tell the dreamer he is doing fine, or to deliver a message to help him live a better life. Most of the time, the message intends to offer psychological support. Is the deceased person coming back from the dead to talk to the dreamer? No one could say. All I can say though is that most of the dreamers who shared this type of dreams strongly felt the tangible presence of the deceased person; they even had clear signs allowing them to identify the deceased one. In the following example, the mutilated hand says it all.

Examples of dreams where we meet a deceased person

My Father

My father is sitting at a small square table in a tavern. Lights are dimmed and the decoration looks like the one in a famous hotel in my city. There is a half full pitcher of beer on the table and my father is holding a glass in his hand. His face has this awkward and caring look so much like him. He is gently moving his mutilated hand, telling us not to worry because he is doing well where he is.

My Partner

I am walking beside Michèle in a hallway in the school where I spent my first grade. I have a feeling of discomfort and nostalgia. I can even smell the odor of the old convent. When getting to another hallway, I see my classroom door. I stop walking and invite Michèle for a visit. She just goes straight ahead and opens a door leading to the outside, telling me she is leaving.

Grief Process Dreams

Grief process dreams tell about our relationships with deceased loved ones. Most often, they show us the way we have yet to go before the grief process can come to an end.

Example of a grief process through three dreams and a ritual

A mother is still grieving the adult daughter she lost five years ago. Through her dreams and a ritual, she will find the courage to work on her grief a very important step for finally starting to live her own life. The current situation, which is being separated from her daughter by an insurmountable roadblock will be stated in the first dream. In the second one, her psychological state will be clearly articulated: She is not ready to let go of her daughter. To help with the process, she deliberately initiates a ritual through a waking dream. A third dream, this time by a close friend of hers, will then confirm her successful efforts. The following describes how this touching process unfolded.

First Dream: The River and the Impassable Waterfall (January)

I had a dream about my daughter Nathalie three days after her birthdate. I am facing a tumultuous river and standing in front of a huge waterfall dividing up into two sections. I cannot possibly reach the other side, because the current would quickly carry me downstream. This waterfall is impassable.

Dreamer's comments

I woke up wondering what this dream meant. I questioned if it had to do with my teaching classes and my training. I ended up convincing myself that the journey was more important than the destination. This dream will take on its full meaning following the third one about the Operating Room, on March 29.

Second Dream: Nathalie (February)

In this dream, I am pregnant with Nathalie. I can feel her presence in a small inner pocket allowing me to track her movements. It feels like a light shape under a piece of fabric, a kind of bag like a kangaroo pouch.

I am getting to the hospital, but it seems like a dangerous place to give birth. Suspicious men are wandering around. Standing upright, I give birth without any help. I am keeping Nathalie into my arms. I tell an attendant, who also looks suspicious, that I will not leave my child with her, because she was still in the womb this morning.

Waking Dream: *The Rainbow* (March 22)

I am going back to meditate at the Richelieu River waterfall in Chambly. It's a beautiful sunny day with a clear sky. Suddenly, I see a rainbow rising above the waterfall, close to the shore. I know this rainbow is a sign. I stare up at it for a long time. I decide to go back home to draw it. Knowing this message relates to Nathalie, I decide to become attentive to any unconscious messages. I suddenly feel the need to set up a small shrine for Nathalie, in the guest room.

I am displaying a photo of Nathalie, fresh flowers and an Angel with broken wings in her glass snow globe on the shrine. Feeling it into my heart, I explain to Nathalie why I am doing this, then I carry her funeral urn away from the room. I put the urn containing her ashes on the shrine. I am crying. I feel peaceful. I then say to Nathalie I healed an old deep wound. In the arms of a therapist, I cried a river and let go of all the anger I had repressed for decades. I tell Nathalie she can go, because I am now able to move forward by myself on my healing journey.

Third Dream: Dreaming about the Operating Room (March 29)

I am standing in an Operating Room. The surgical procedure aims to **cut the ties**. *The head of the OR tells me that nine nurses are available and that the team members for the procedure are a friend of mine, my therapist and myself. Upon waking up, I am told that our mission is accomplished, and Nathalie can cross over to the other side of the world.*

Dreamer's comments

This is where the dream about the waterfall took on its full meaning; the impassable waterfall reflected the two worlds, my own and Nathalie's, the one she came from and where she went back.

So, I was able to write down the following message for Nathalie. "My love, when the time comes for me to leave my body behind, I will get back to you. We will be together forever and our love will last for eternity". I asked for a sign proving she had set out on the journey back home.

A close friend had a dream she told me about, without knowing about the Operating Room dream (procedure for cutting the ties). She dreamed I had set up a photo collage of all Nathalie's photos displayed till now in a showcase at home. In her dream, I had replaced all photos in the showcase with ones from my youngest daughter and my granddaughter. I had given their proper place to the people staying with me in this world.

It became absolutely clear to me that Nathalie used a messenger through dreams to tell me she had crossed over to the other world, and I had to dedicate myself to the loved ones in my current life from now on.

Resolution Dreams

Resolution dreams are similar to nightmares except that they bring a resolution to a problem outlined in the dream. As a result, the dreamer wakes up without intense feelings of terror, panic or impending danger. On the contrary, he knows upon waking up he successfully escaped a very difficult situation. The dream generally draws an analogy with a waking life situation the dreamer was able to avoid, recently attempted to solve or will find a way to resolve through the solution symbolically depicted in the dream. This dream type has both a self-regulating function and a support function.

Example of a resolution dream

A Near Plane Crash

I am aboard an aircraft and I am doing fine. We are preparing for landing. The landing is hard, and there is turmoil at the tail of the aircraft. A few women are screaming with fear. Nevertheless, everything is going well. The aircraft almost comes to a stop but it suddenly starts to climb again. I do not understand why the pilot is initiating a climb and as the plane is climbing up, I can see another aircraft on my left blowing out of the sky. I realise the debris could have been potentially dangerous on the runway and that's probably why the pilot initiated a climb (as if knowing in advance another aircraft would blow out of the sky). That decision might also have been taken because of some hazardous conditions at the airport.

The aircraft is flying at very low altitude, and at the last minute build-ings looking very gloomy and dark become visible. The pilot narrowly avoids a collision with the buildings and big power lines.

The plane finally lands safely and I find myself handling a heavy suitcase at the airport, dragging it along down the stairs. I see a mother holding her baby in her arms. It looks like the elevators are out of service following this disturbing event. I am unhappy about the situation and I wake up.

Dreamer's comments

I had this dream one month after going abroad for a writing project. I actually got on a plane, but nothing tragic occurred. At the airport, I had to drag a heavy suitcase down the stairs though. After arriving abroad, I experienced some kind of crashing, since I felt overwhelmed and very tired. I feared I would be unable to get my energy back (no elevator). The mother holding her child symbolises my writing project.

For me, the existential message is as follows. The dream is telling me I avoided some pitfalls (aircraft blowing out of the sky, gloomy looking buildings and power lines) by taking care of myself, and a worst scenario was averted since there was no plane crash. In addition, my energy level gradually went back up. Since the elevator is inoperative in the dream, I feel it means I have to make the elevator operational again by taking time to restore my energy level and to take care of myself before going back to work on my writing project. I resolved the situation by taking good care of myself, and I realised the message should be a reminder.

Resources Dreams

In a resources dream, the "I" in the dreamer or another character in the dream resolves a situation by using one's own resources. The dream's function is to give the dreamer access to a new resource or to point out he recently acquired it. While this dream type is similar to a resolution dream, it differs in the proactive attitude of the dreamer – or another character in the dream – who figures out how to act directly on the problem outlined in the dream.

Example of a resources dream: A 65-year-old person had the following dream

A Swimming Lesson in Ice Cold Water

In my dream, I have a swimming lesson in a pool filled with ice cold water and large chunks of ice. There is about 10 beginners or advanced students. It seems to me my own daughter is also part of the group. I am wearing a heavy wetsuit made of black plastic material and I do not

know if this heavy outfit will enable me to stay afloat. The teacher is asking us to do an exercise in the deep end of the swimming pool and to even go beneath the ice. I am afraid of this. The other beginners do not feel secure either. So, I say to the teacher "I am leaving this class. It's for advanced students, not for beginners. I don't even have to be here, and I don't take pleasure in this class".

Through her dreamwork, the dreamer realised she must put an end to a specific situation in her life she finds both unsuitable and unpleasant. Above all, she understood it is right to make choices taking into account if she has fun or not. She can choose what suits her. In this case, the conscious "I" is reinforced, and the identity strengthened by experiencing a clear and straightforward self-expression in the dream.

Validation Dreams

In a validation dream, often similar to a clear dream, the dreamer is reassured that his decision, his perception or his feeling about a situation is right. Since this dream type essentially has a psychological support function, the existential message will not bring anything new, but will validate a decision or direction the dreamer foresaw in his waking life.

Example of a validation dream: A young fiancée had the following dream

Getting Married

In my dream, I am getting married and I am not feeling well. I think something is wrong, I do have doubts and getting married with Jean does not feel comfortable. Then it suddenly comes up to my mind I am not getting married with Jean, but rather with Mario! So, everything is fine.

The young fiancée's dream ended with this and she felt released upon waking up. She had the same dream time and again, every couple of months. It was featuring different partners each time, usually ex-boyfriends, and had the same ending. This young woman got married 30 years ago and never questioned her choice ever since. The dream stopped repeating after getting married.

Creative Dreams

In a creative dream, something creative gets accomplished: A story unfolds night after night, inspiring contents for a novel or a painting, a drawing or an original musical work the dreamer will recreate while awake. Its most obvious function is to foster creative expression. In many cases, the creative subject matter has a symbolic value from which the dreamer can learn an existential message. For example, if you are playing music in a dream and go on performing it in your waking life, chances are you will be able to feel what is being expressed through the music, and possibly identify some aspect of your life experience that went unnoticed.

Example of a creative dream

The Fashion Show

I am attending a fashion show featuring beautiful and very stylish dresses. One dress in particular draws my attention, as its shimmering fabric looks like a rainbow.

Dreamer's comments

About once a year, I have a dream about a fashion show featuring amazing but always distinctive dresses. I wake up every time with a strong urge to draw them and to create a high fashion collection, because I find them so attractive. I never created and probably will never create such a collection. When drawing those dream dresses however, I realise they reflect a shift in identity year after year, as if pointing to a new self-image from time to time.

Healing Dreams

Healing dreams are particularly fascinating, and examples are found in many books. For example, a sick person sees in a dream a doctor, a wise man or a friend suggesting a specific medication or treatment, and it brings instant recovery. Cases were identified where the dreamer does something that brings his own complete recovery or is able to cure someone else (see Garfield, 1991, 1983).

Example of a healing dream: A 40-year-old teacher and linguist had the following dream

Rats

I am in a house similar to the place where I live. I live with Denise, a friend of mine. We are surrounded by rats going around quite naturally. The rats do not fill me with disgust. We are even cooking food with rat meat in a big pot. This scene does not seem horrible to me at all. Denise and I are both feeling good.

Excerpt from the Dreamer's Dream Journal

Upon waking up, it did not feel like a nightmare, but I felt bad for dreaming about rats. I hate rats in real life. I think they are both ugly and disgusting. I am definitely convinced this dream is important though.

While feeling an urge to analyze and work on the dream in a group, I also felt ashamed of myself for having this dream. I finally took the risk to share my dream. To embrace it even more, I decided to use clay and I almost magically sculpted three rats. The first one was unsophisticated, primitive and rude; the second one was more sophisticated with a clean-cut look, and finally the third one was very stylish.

Dreamwork helped me remember my son's accident in Switzerland when he suffered eye injuries. For me, the first rat represented how ugly my son's eye looked following the accident. After the initial shock, I quickly found out my son had a strong ability to recover and the feeling of ugliness progressively went away. My son's eye looked increasingly better and the scar faded away. It looked more and more refined, just like the second and third rats in my dream. Sculpting the three rats with clay helped me embracing all of this, feeling self-empowered and, in a more powerful way, understanding I had power over my son's healing. I could sculpt my son's eye again, just like I had sculpted the third rat turning it into a beautiful one through my hands.

Comments

This dream has an unquestionable value, as it showed clearly to a mother how she could help her son. She started sculpting her son's eye by channeling energy through her hands. The dream enabled her to acknowledge her ability for hands-on healing and to empower herself. The therapeutic value of this power commands respect, although it cannot be scientifically proven. Nevertheless, her son recovered much faster than medical doctors could ever have anticipated.

Incubation Dreams

Through these dreams, we find a solution to a problem we have been struggling with for a long time. Scientific discoveries sometimes get revealed the same way about something the dreamer thought about for a long time. These situations create the conditions specific to "incubation".

On the other hand, we can deliberately cause incubation by programming a specific dream. For this purpose, the dreamer just needs to go to bed with a specific intention in mind and to repeat it several times in a relaxed state. This technique will be addressed in more detail in Chapter 3, which deals with brief dreamwork methods. For now, you only need to know different types of dreams can be programmed this way, whether they are creative, healing, lucid or telepathic ones, etc.

Therefore, the incubation dream's function is to respond to a conscious desire for solving a problem, for healing or understanding oneself, as well as for inducing a creative endeavor or reaching any other stated objective.

Example of an incubation dream

I had the following dream when one of my past love relationships was highly unsatisfactory. The time spent with my boyfriend had been difficult and I went to bed asking for clarifications about what was going through my night dreams.

The Swan With Burned-Off Wings

My boyfriend and I are grilling birds on a hibachi grill outdoors. I can see the head, the body, the neck and the wings of the three birds being grilled. The bird whose head I can see is still alive; three quarters of its wings are burned and brownish. It flies away and comes back, landing on the hibachi grill resignedly with its head down, unable to fly.

Dreamer's comments

Following this dream, I decided to draw the resigned bird giving it wings to fly. I instantly felt better. It looked like a beautiful gracious swan (the dream's title was inspired by this). The meaning of my dream and the answer to my question became clear while drawing the bird. Having just signed a contract for a job in the town my boyfriend lived in, it meant I would be living with him. I had made a decision failing to take into account how difficult our relationship was. Through the dream, I was informed that with the signing of this paper, my wings were burned off and the freedom I needed was taken away. I had made a bad decision. Later on, through a combination of circumstances, I ended up being released from my commitment. And a few months later, I finally faced the fact that this love relationship was not nurturing.

This incubation dream fulfilled its function by providing me with a much-needed answer. As for the drawing inspired by the dream, it had a therapeutic function since I started feeling much better after giving new wings to the bird I drew.

Transpersonal Dreams

In a transpersonal dream, archetypes coming from the collective unconscious emerge. Jung introduced the collective unconscious concept, a kind of psychological legacy shared among human beings which is composed of pre-existing patterns in the psyche. These determine the components of the so-called objective psyche; they are universally present and repeated in each individual at birth. The collective unconscious is structured by the archetypes (Lévesque, 2010). Robert A. Johnson, an American Jungian analyst, defines archetypes as follows:

> [...] the characteristic patterns that pre-exist in the collective psyche of the human race that repeat themselves eternally in the psyches of individual human beings and determine the basic ways that we perceive and function as psychological beings (1986, p. 27).

In other words, archetypes are symbols relating to the general human experience and found in the collective unconscious shared by each of us, regardless of our particular experiences. These symbols, along with the purely personal ones, emerge in many different ways from our imaginary and in our dreams in particular. It is very important to know how to identify a transpersonal dream, because archetypes arising from it can be extremely positive or negative. If the archetypes are positive, breathing life into symbols through a drawing or a dialogue (see Chapters 4 and 5) allows a positive transformation. If they are negative, dreamwork through a brief method is more appropriate, especially an approach aiming to change the ending of the dream (see Chapter 3), since their huge potential for negative energy is worth transforming into positive energy. In contrast, personal negative symbols must be worked on and understood. Robert A. Johnson (1986) helps us drawing a distinction between purely personal symbols and archetypes, the latter being often presented by the unconscious as divine, royal, magical or mythical images.

Examples of negative archetypes are images of the devil, of a dragon, of a bloodthirsty emperor, etc. A personal negative symbol would rather look like a monster hostilely chasing you, a character intending to kill you, a thief etc. What is the difference between the two? The archetype is always a collective image, which means it can be found in art, culture, myths or tales. In other words, the image has a universal attribute applicable to each human being's life experience.

The function of these dreams apparently is to point the way forward to pursue one's growth or to indicate what would be the wrong way to go if one is dealing with a negative archetype. This type of dream often marks a step on the spiritual and personal growth of an individual. While the dreamer may not be aware of it beforehand, such a dream can be life changing (Bulkeley, 2000, in Pesant and Zadra, 2010).

Example of a transpersonal dream: A 30-year-old Native American woman had the following dream

White Bison Lady

In my dream, I am seeing through a window a rat with eyes going on and off like flashing lights. Every time its eyes close, the rat vanishes. I find it troubling. I point it out to other people around me, but nobody can see it. I am the only one who sees it …

As my friend Anne comes in, I try to tell her about the rat incident, but nobody is listening, and they all treat me like I am crazy. But Anne knows in fact. I am crying, I am feeling afraid and I am thinking about the rat, being sure it will come back.

I am sure it will get in; I can fathom it. If it comes in, I will have to kill it. Then I realise I won't, as the rat might intend to help me go further and I shouldn't be afraid of it.

I now see through the window a deer, a bear, a hare and many other animals going by. All of a sudden, I see Native American men on horses running in the same direction.

I watch them go by. Anne is looking at me and tells me I am called upon by White Bison Lady. She is crying because she "knows". I ask her if I should be afraid and what I should do about it. Anne tells me it can be quite scary, but it depends on how I respond.

Comments

The dreamer is a woman who works in clay, carving magnificent and complex animal figures tangled up with characters, and all this magically comes out of her artistic hands. She is just starting to acknowledge her own artistic talent and to be devoted to art. Often being the only one to *see what she sees,* she has a lot of fears and hesitations, as her talent is rather unique. Saying yes to her talent implies accepting the existential solitude coming from having something unique to offer; it also means sharing her vision instead of being *the only one who sees,* and this choice in itself is a dilemma. *White Bison Lady* is a very important spiritual figure in the legends of the Native American Sioux people (Sams & Carson, 1988). White Bison Lady is calling her to follow her own path, to give shape to her Native American Spirit through art and to stop being afraid, since *it depends on how she responds,* as her friend said. Therefore, the dream highlights the direction for her personal, spiritual and artistic development.

Paranormal Dreams

Premonitory dreams, telepathic dreams and clairvoyant dreams are included in this category. One common feature they all share is to include information delivered to the dreamer through paranormal channels, which means outside the normal communication channels, in other words the senses. In the current state of scientific knowledge, there are no explanations on how this information in conveyed to the dreamer, even if these phenomena do exist. The purpose of these dreams is to provide information not readily accessible.

Premonitory Dreams

As suggested by its name, a premonitory dream reveals forthcoming events. No one knows for sure if a dream is premonitory until the predicted future events are witnessed. Most of the premonitory dreams involve people with whom we have established very close relationships. However, people having such fine powers can even dream of persons who are not close relations or of distant circumstances. If you are dreaming about the death of a loved one for example, is it predicting a real-life event or is it something else? Most of the time, this type of dream is symbolic and delivers a personal message rather than a premonition.

Few people frequently have premonitory dreams. Those who have frequent ones have developed skills allowing them to identify such dreams given the particular impressions left upon waking up, or the specific signs associated with them.

Premonitory dreams often feature events to come with great accuracy and detail, just as depicted in the dream. Nevertheless, circumstances might be very different as shown in the following example.

Example of a premonitory dream: A 30-year-old woman had the following dream

A Romantic Date

I am going on a romantic date at a sidewalk café in Old Québec with a couple of friends and a man I have never met. With an injured left leg, I am slow and afraid I am going to miss my date.

I am walking across the Plains of Abraham and it feels like I am going down a flight of wooden stairs. Halfway down, there are no more steps. There is a steep slope with rocks on it.

Then I notice my friends and the unknown man are watching the time and looking all around for me. Chantal comes to meet me, asking me why I am late and making it clear their friend is impatient to meet me ... I wake up right away.

Comments

By working on her dream in a therapy group, the dreamer became aware she was still emotionally hurting from a previous love relationship which prevented opening up to a new one. Shortly after this dream, she met the man who was with her friends in the dream, someone she had never met before, and they started a love relationship! Needless to say, she reacted very strongly when she first met him. Therefore, the dream allowed her to look upon him as a potential love partner. Had it not been for her dream, her inner wounds might have prevented her from recognising this potential relationship.

Telepathic Dreams

In a telepathic dream, there is some kind of thought transference between the dreamer and another person. These dreaming experiences are commonly covered in literature. For example, a dreamer had a dream where a close one came to say goodbye or to deliver an important message, and in the morning the news broke that the loved one had passed away. This type of dream, which is also a *dream about death*, seems to allow for communication between two beings. Telepathic dreams can also allow for real-time communication between two dreamers, as in a *shared dream*. Linda Magallòn, dream educator and research expert in lucid dreaming and abnormal dreams, and Barbara Shor, also dream educator, both define shared dreams as follows: "In shared dreams, two or more dreamers apparently come together in the same dream landscape and experience similar events" (Magallòn and Shor, in Krippner, 1991).

They both include in their definition a voluntary element: the shared dream is in fact planned within a group. I think this does not necessarily fit into the definition of this dream type. A shared dream might as well occur spontaneously between two or many dreamers.

Example of a shared dream

Sun Bear and the Sun Wheel

I am assembling a Sun Wheel[2] with my partner. I am using metal or rubber rods for the wheel spokes. The wheel cannot be completed because we do not have enough spokes. I go and see Sun Bear who is also creating a Sun Wheel with his wife Wabun. Sun Bear provides for the missing rods, cut just about the right length. The landscape is in poor condition and barren, without any plant cover, and the only visible houses are two wood cabins made of used planks.

Dreamer's comments

The following morning, I shared my dream with my partner and found out he had the same one, except for the rods. They were bamboo sticks. He was also creating a Sun Wheel with me. Did we communicate telepathically? Or with Sun Bear? The context might be insightful since my partner and I had this dream after a workshop with Sun Bear, a Native American Shaman. We had not assembled a Sun Wheel yet, but this concept was familiar to us. Over the weekend, Sun Bear had mentioned he was often communicating with people through dreams. Was this a simple suggestion? Such explanatory hypotheses

---

2 For Native American people, a "Sun Wheel" or "Medicine Wheel" is a stone circle with four or seven stones in the center and twelve stones on the circumference. Cardinal points can be represented in the wheel. It usually does not come with spokes.

should not be ruled out. However, having the same dream remains troubling, considering the only difference was the material sticks/rods were made from.

Clairvoyant Dreams

In these dreams, by some mysterious process, the dreamer seems to perceive catastrophic events actually occurring while he is dreaming. However, it is difficult to prove that the dreamer's perception occurred simultaneously with the events taking place.

A clairvoyant dream gives access to information not readily available. But how is this possible? I am assuming that the external events perceived by the dreamer through a clairvoyant dream echo and resonate with an inner process, thus the events resonate with him. While some dreamers have an amazing capability for clairvoyant perception, others are totally insensitive to this kind of experience. Currently unknown variables could very well take part in these phenomena.

Example of a clairvoyant dream

The following example is from an article by a Norwegian man, Mr Jon Tolaas (1991). It is about a young 22-year-old woman who had a dream about an avalanche which resulted in a number of deaths. The next morning, being sure the event occurred in real life, she turned on the radio to confirm whether it actually happened. There was indeed a major avalanche that caused many deaths. After contemplating natural explanations for such an apparently clairvoyant perception, Jon Tolaas discovered many possibilities. The dreamer could have heard weather forecasts about a forthcoming avalanche, paying little attention to it; she might also be used to weather conditions prevailing before an avalanche and felt these without even realising it.

He also made another assumption, a quite interesting one. He assumed there was "dream sensing" and explained that the dreamer could have been subliminally exposed to infrasonic vibrations typically associated with volcanic eruptions, earthquakes, landslides or other seismic activity. This assumption would be worth investigating before concluding it is a clairvoyant dream. Research will eventually shed some light on these phenomena. Regardless, Tolaas did not rule out the possibility that this particular case was an extrasensory clairvoyance phenomenon.

Lucid Dreams

During a lucid dream, while the dreamer knows he is dreaming, he has also a very clear sense he is sleeping. A lucid dream should not be confused with those times when we are not completely awake. In this type of dream, you can make a decision to respond the way you choose to what is happening, since you know you are dreaming. You can even choose to explore issues present in your waking life, for example to go and meet persons you are in a dispute with.

These dreams leave a very strong impression, a feeling we are mastering our destiny, even in our waking life. When appearing in your dreaming life, these dreams mark the beginning of greater self-consciousness, which is a function specific to this dream type.

Lucid dreams being a very special experience, they will be addressed in Chapter 6.

Example of a lucid dream: A 30-year-old man had the following dream

Native American land: A Journey across Stark Dark Waters

I want to go to desert lands mostly owned by Native American people. As I turn my attention to a military map (a very detailed one), I notice the boundaries defining the state lands reserved for Native American people. I am also aware that getting caught in these territories could mean death, since they are considered as Sacred Land. I must ask permission from the Native American people. I make up my mind, realising it is the right way and the best way to do it, although I could be denied access. And what about offering something in return? It is dangerous, but I have a strong desire to visit these Native people lands since I am fascinated with them.

The situation is shifting. I am now on a boat navigating on a stark dark sea, looking for Native American lands. Something massive is pushing the vessel that keeps rolling and pitching. I know it is a whale playing with us (the vessel and I). The whale is pushing the vessel and I can feel its stark black massive body in the water. Being sick and tired of the whale's actions, I realise "Why not leaving now?" That is when I become aware that I can take action and change this situation by flying high in the sky, and go wherever I want to. Still being under the impression I am on the vessel with the whale, I am now wandering around a room. As I leap and walk through the wall, it liquefies and turns into various colorful inks, mainly bright yellow and red. It looks like crumbly acrylic paint. Every time I touch the walls or the ceiling, everything is liquefying. I become more and more aware I am dreaming. I walk into the room and as I turn the corner, I am about to access a room I am not familiar with. At the same time, I am becoming more and more aware of being awake in the dream, and of the bedroom where I am sleeping. This state remained for a few more seconds and then I found it more and more difficult to stay lucid. I woke up.

Excerpt from the Dreamer's Journal

Coming out of this dream, I am still holding the feeling I can fly and go wherever I want, and especially walk through walls and ceilings which turn into a liquefied state. I realise that my decision to face the Native American people's

reactions triggered the awareness of being in a dream. Subsequently, the feeling of being sick and tired of the whale's actions had the same impact. I enjoy realising that my active consciousness yields spectacular results like turning walls and ceilings into multicolored inks. I also enjoy feeling I can influence the outcome of the dream. I am not striving to change everything I want, but I appreciate having a substantial impact through the decisions I make. On the other hand, I keep feeling frustrated about not having visited the Native American lands. I somehow had become embroiled in the pleasure of exercising power over the dream's scenario without realising I had lost sight of the objective I was initially pursuing. I am also becoming aware I can reach different levels of lucidity during a dream.

Comments

In this case, the dreamer became aware he was empowered to act, and this awareness remained even after waking up, enabling him to see himself as more and more responsible for his choices and his future. He faced a frequent obstacle specific to lucid dreaming: He became embroiled in the pleasure of having control over the dream's scenario and lost sight of the objective he was initially pursuing. There comes a time in one's self-growth, – whether in dreams or in real life – when one should let go of the fun to exercise power to make room for a more important goal. In other words, the ego must make way for the Self, in a Jungian sense.

Prelucid Dreams

As its name implies, a prelucid dream is one where the dreamer is nearly lucid. For example, the dreamer may know he is dreaming or be aware of an impossible event or of a different reality, without finding a way to act or influence the situation. It might be that the lucidity condition lasts just a few seconds as if the dreamer can figure out that he is dreaming without becoming aware of the opportunities he has, or that the lucid state cannot be maintained more than a few seconds. Needless to say, a prelucid dream can lead to a lucid dream since it includes hints the dreamer can learn to identify.

Example of a prelucid dream

The Pile of Rock

I am looking at a weird dark landscape both barren and desert, with black rock. Scattered here and there, piles of rocks in the shape of human hands point the way. It is foggy and it's hard to see things clearly. In my dream, I realise that what I am contemplating is the deer's world whose meat I ate last night, and that is why this landscape seems unfamiliar to me. It feels like I am in a portal between two universes.

Dreamer's comments

This dream is a prelucid one for it contains real-life elements: I ate deer meat the night before. Furthermore, I am aware – although not fully – that I am dreaming. On the other hand, I can consider the dream as a symbolic one and search for its meaning: I am exploring within me a new universe remaining unclear yet. I actually sense I am between two universes and while I feel as though I am surrounded by fog, I can see markers (piles of rocks) which prevent me from feeling completely lost. I acknowledge it is true in real life also. Painting a picture of my path, showing where I am and how I feel, the dream has a self-regulating function.

Recurring Dreams

A recurring dream is a dreaming scene that keeps coming back as it is or almost unchanged, at more or less regular intervals. This type of dream is particularly important since it keeps bringing up the same existential message time and again, probably because the dreamer has not understood it yet. A recurring dream illustrates a psychic evolution over an extended period of time. Widely known examples include dreams where one is falling down, ends up paralyzed or keeps seeing the same nightmare scenario.

Example of a recurring dream: A 90-year-old lady shared the following dream. It kept coming back over 20 years. It started when she was 20 years old and ended when she was in her forties

A Search on a Road

In my dream, I am walking on the road close to our own farm and to my grandfather's house. I am looking for something, not knowing exactly what. I wake up after a while. Later in life, I will dream I am back on the same road, and for all the subsequent dreams, I will pick up from where I left off in the previous one. It lasted for years and years.

Eventually, I get to the end of the road, close to the mountain. It feels like I am walking around it. At one spot, rocks look like they were cut. Stuck in the rock, a building made of large and thick wooden planks looks like an old chapel. I walk into that building, looking for something and get pebbles and loose boards out of the way. I find a piece of white paper with words on it; I remember only one word in some old print: Ego. I know this is not what I am looking for. Then I step on a broken wooden plank and surprisingly, it can easily be lifted off. Underneath, I find a moccasin with small change and I know it is not what I am looking for either. I step on another loose board, lift it off and find the body of Father Warry underneath. In the old times, he was selling remedies and had been in the newspapers. He is dead but he looks alive with red cheeks and eyes wide open. I have found what I am looking for. This dream stopped recurring after finding Father Warry's body.

Comments

This dream is a great example of the individuation process described by Carl Jung. Jung (1993) states that in the first stage of life the ego builds up and becomes the core structure of the personality, whereas in middle life, the Self, or spiritual side, becomes central. I think this recurring dream illustrates this quest for the Self, which is confirmed by some elements; the dreamer effectively finds the *Ego* first and knows intuitively it is not what she is looking for. Furthermore, the building looks like an old chapel and the character is a religious figure. Finally, spiritual life was always very important for this lady and prayer has always been a part of her life. It is interesting to note that when I first met her, I asked her if she knew what is meant by the word "ego" and she did not know. What a significant example of the broad knowledge of the unconscious remaining unknown or buried by the conscious mind! And this knowledge can be accessed through our night dreams.

Dream Series

Recurring symbols or images sometimes come back in various dreams of a quite different nature. They constitute a series of dreams to be used to understand one's psychic growth. Their function is to illustrate one's evolution.

Example of a series of dreams: A 38-year-old woman working as a helping relationship professional had the following series of dreams over a four-month span

The Snake in Clear Water

My feet and my legs are soaking in shallow waters in the lake. I lift the skirt of my long dress so that it does not get wet. All of a sudden, a thin black snake appears in the clear waters of the lake. I get frightened and rush out of the water.

A Snake Bite on My Left Leg

A snake bites my left leg and is moving up my pants. I grab it and get rid of it. I am waiting, wondering if it's poisonous. Feeling my leg get numb, I start screaming "The snake is poisonous, let's go to the hospital".

The Python

My 14-year-old niece is holding in her arms a huge green snake with scales. It looks like a python. Considering it is too big for her, I ask her to go and leave it in my bedroom.

Facing the Black Snake

I am tied up in the center of some space. I see a small black snake on my left. I know for sure he is going to bite me. I feel terrified. However, I decide to face it and allow myself to feel terrified by it without waking up.

Zeus' Finger

*Like the one in Michelangelo's painting, Zeus throws a lightning bolt with his finger and it penetrates my third eye. At that moment, the word **empowerment** comes to my mind.*

Excerpt from the Dreamer's Journal

At one point in my personal journey, I was on a quest for the right to sexual pleasure. Although my sexual life was actually gratifying, I still felt some detrimental restrictions concerning sexual pleasure. The growing presence of snakes in this series of dreams indicates a need for a complete conquest of my sexual life is emerging strongly. Needless to say, it is frightening for me since I am so afraid "I rush out of the water"; "I feel pain" and "My left leg gets numb". I even feel terrified. However, through my dream explorations as well as in my waking life, I can face terror. In the final dream afterwards, female power penetrates through a lightning bolt (empowerment). At first glance, I did not consider this last dream as being part of the whole series; however, when trying to understand it through dreamwork, I saw similarities between the strong power from the lightning bolt through my third eye and the venom from the snake biting my left leg and going up, which was also powerful. On the other hand, I saw similarities between those two images and the intensity of an orgasm.

Beyond sexuality, this series of dreams is about my emotional needs as a whole. After the final dream, I felt more and more able to take action in order to satisfy my emotional needs, to ask for what I need and to accept getting in touch with my emotional or sexual needs instead of denying them.

Comments

In this dream, the Zeus figure is a fascinating one, since this god is the ultimate symbol of the father. Ultimately, it is through the father figure that a young woman is able to conquer her female power during her psychological/sexual development. While her father confirms she is entitled to sexuality by making her feel how desirable she is, he is also directing her toward other partners than himself to satisfy her needs. The dream is confirming what this process means and that some resolving occurred, since the young woman successfully conquered her female power.

Comments on Chapter 1

I never cease to be amazed at how dreams are rich, diversified and complex. In addition, dream types are numerous and have multiple functions. As for the existential messages, they are never-ending. Dreams offer a whole world to be explored as well as a wealth of information and insights that will never run dry.

Through the different types of dreams and their multiple functions, the unconscious is always collaborating with the conscious mind to give it further information and help it to get control over the inner world. Working on dreams is about honoring this input and asking the conscious mind to collaborate with the unconscious in return.

In the next chapter, you will learn how to successfully keep a Dream Journal, which will enable you to draw knowledge from your dream life. Before going further, I would invite you to create your own dream dictionary. Dreams reflect a significantly individualised reality. As a matter of fact, there can be significant differences in the meaning of symbols from a person to another, and their meaning can even vary with the various life stages in someone's life. After a while, you will notice that some dream images or symbols keep returning. These images can be used to create your own personal dream dictionary; please note any specific meaning associated with them for each dream in which they emerge. Series of dreams are particularly rich in this regard. You will also notice your symbols show identical or similar meanings. However, please be mindful that the meaning of a symbol can vary according to life circumstances and your personal journey. Also keep in mind that you should never take for granted the meaning of a symbol from one dream to another.

2

How to Keep a Dream Journal

Keeping a Dream Journal is a fascinating endeavor, but it is time consuming and interior willingness is required. You will eventually set your own pace both for writing down your dreams and finding the existential message. You do not necessarily need to write down your dreams every day or to work on each of them. On the contrary, it would be too demanding to use them all as a tool for growth. Keeping your Dream Journal must be fun.

Please let me suggest a particular approach for keeping a Dream Journal. Using two pages, first write down the dream itself as well as some information on the left page, then use the right page to elucidate the dream's message (See example at the end of this chapter). After reading this chapter, you will be all set to start a Dream Journal.

But first of all, many people who have difficulty remembering their dreams are looking for ways to do it. See the summary box at the end of this chapter to learn how.

Left Page of the Dream Journal: The Dream Story

On the left side of your Dream Journal, in addition to noting the dream's description, I would recommend to write down specific notes about your dream in order to facilitate tracking and classification of data (see example of a Dream Journal at the end of this chapter). These notes will make some elements stand out from your series of Dream Journals, for example the most common dream types, personal existential issues, any recurring images and dreams and where you stand in your psychological evolution.

Included in your notes will be the dream number, the date, the dream type, the title, the existential message, the significant or recurring images and recent life events. It might seem a lot of work, but writing down this information will prove to be absolutely worthwhile, since they allow maximum use of your dream material in the short, medium and long terms. Having experimented myself a broad range of methods, I found out that keeping my Dream Journal this way proved to be very gratifying.

Let's now see the implication and the rationale behind including notes on the left side of the Dream Journal.

Numbering a Dream

This information is very useful for the purpose of tracking some elements. For example, if you want the recurring image of your childhood home to stand out of your whole set of dreams, you can simply take note of the number of each dream in which it occurs. Ideally include the current year followed with the dream number. Thus, 2020–1 refers to the first dream you wrote down in 2020. It is important for the year to be included, since your Dream Journal might sooner or later spread out over many years, and be comprised of many notebooks. Specifying the year will make it easier for you to sort things out in all your Dream Journals. Writing down the dream number in the top right corner will allow to easily sort out to which dream a page relates.

Setting a Date

Of course, the date is an important piece of information in terms of the timeframe of a dream. When re-reading the content of a dream, especially if you remember the events that took place in your waking life back then, or you jotted them down, you could possibly understand the existential message that might have slipped through at that time. For example, a few years ago, I had a very clear dream about my psychological circumstances. Yet, it was not until much later I realised its extent, after reading it again.

The Dream Type

It could be useful to know about a classification of the different dream types so that you can identify each dream type and take note of it. Such a classification is included in the first chapter, but you could also make your own one based on your dreams.

If you take note of each dream type, you could for example review all seemingly premonitory dreams over a year in order to check if they came true, or to point out lucid dreams, healing dreams, etc. You could also highlight the different types of dreams using a set of color pencils. This way, while browsing through your Dream Journal, you would quickly identify the dreams that stand out from the symbolic ones, the most common type.

The Existential Message

It will be possible to unveil the dream's message only after having worked on it one way or the other using the right page of the Dream Journal.

However, please write the existential message on the left page, following the dream type, to make sure it will be easily accessible for future reference. This section will often be left empty though, since you will not work on all dreams.

So, after elucidating the message of a dream using the right page, please take time to word the message in a clear and concise sentence, and write it down in the appropriate section on the left side. It will be more impactful and more efficient if it is clear and brief.

What the Existential Message is

For Frederick Perls (1972), a famous Gestalt psychiatrist, each dream delivers a message about the dreamer's life. As for me, all dreams deliver such a message, except for the premonitory ones. Furthermore, the message is never trivial but highly important for the dreamer's waking life. The purpose of almost all methods proposed in this book is to discover the existential message by way of some dreamwork from which an inner certitude arises, rather than trying to find a rational explanation for the dream. Finding the existential message is thus a core aspect of any dreamwork. Considering it might seem like a difficult task to identify it clearly, let's use some examples from the previous chapter, followed with explanations about how the existential message can be discovered or identified.

- Dream from a grandmother – Going back to the convent
  This grandmother understood that going out with her friends is very important to her, that she misses it when she does not do it and that such occasions make her feel like she is recapturing her youth.
- A healing dream – The rats
  The mother understood she had power over her situation and could contribute to her son's healing.
- One of my incubation dreams – The swan with burned off wings
  Making the decision to start living with my boyfriend was a bad one, considering the love relationship was not nurturing.
- A lucid dream – Native American land, a journey across stark dark waters
  The dreamer understood he was empowered to take action and could have an impact on reality on his own will, and that he was responsible for his choices and his future.

Discovering the Existential Message of Dreams

Many people find this step particularly difficult. Yet, the existential message emerges all by itself through the dreamwork. Without dreamwork, the message you will decode will be at best an assumption or a spontaneous association in your mind. Since the existential message is the last step for each proposed method, the message will naturally emerge as a conclusion arising from the previous steps.

You can identify the existential message by asking yourself what is left from your dreamwork or what is being taught or revealed by the dream as a whole. You might easily get carried away with endless speculations if you review every element in a dream in search of a message. On the contrary, it is easier to give attention to the dream as a whole rather than to its various elements. If many existential messages come to your mind, find out the global message that encompasses them all.

The key to the message is the feeling arising from the previous steps and what stirred a reaction in you, whether positive or negative; the initial meaning that comes to your mind is not necessarily the answer.

Pitfalls to Avoid

Robert A. Johnson (2009/1986) identifies two possible pitfalls when trying to identify the existential message. He refers to this as the "interpretation". He suggests avoiding this:

- Any interpretation that would tend to unnecessarily *inflate* your ego. If you see yourself making an interpretation where you are *peacocking* and applauding yourself for being so wonderful and superior to other mortals, then this interpretation is incorrect;
- Interpretations that take away your responsibility. It might be very tempting to take advantage of dreams to blame other persons for the events in our lives … These interpretations do not only lead to complacency about oneself, they usually are inaccurate and psychologically irrelevant.

In my own view, it is important to avoid these two pitfalls. Another pitfall would be to confuse "existential message" with "moral conscience" or "blaming". A dream is not intended to flatter one's ego nor to break down or criticise oneself. It gives some *insight into* one's inner world by demonstrating symbolically what is going on, just like a movie.

Identifying an Existential Message

An existential message has the following characteristics:

- It gives the impression that we discovered something new about us and our life;
- It makes us feel like our development towards personal well-being is reinforced by showing the way forward or the decision to take;
- It gives hope;
- It often brings relief;
- It comes as a surprise, precisely because it is revealing something new;
- Or on the contrary, it confirms in a stronger way what we had intuited;
- It summarises our general understanding of the dream.

In each proposed method, the last step involves bringing an existential message to light. You can refer to this section each time you need help to discover an existential message, until you understand clearly what it is all about and how to discover it.

The Dream's Title

Giving a title to a dream can be very delightful! It feels like taking ownership of the dream and pulling out the key image to make it the most important part of the title. A clear wording is all that is needed to recall the dream and its atmosphere.

The Dream's Story

To give a vibrant description of a dream, it is important to follow two instructions:

- First, the dream should be worded in the present tense as though you are actually dreaming – for example, "I am dreaming about a walk in the woods ..."
- Second, always state where *you* are in the dream: For example, "I am on a mountain with many friends" would be a preferable wording instead of "They are" or "We are". As you may have guessed, the "I" is the important point here. If you are not a character in the dream, at least relate what is taking place "I am dreaming about this scene ..."

These two instructions from the Gestalt approach (See Perls, 1992) have the effect of bringing back the intensity and atmosphere specific to a dream because they imply taking ownership. The prevailing impression felt upon waking up is recalled instantly when writing down a dream this way. This is definitely how the dream's essence can be grasped.

I found out about another very interesting way to narrate my dreams and I occasionally use it. Rather than providing a chronological sequence of events, I start with wording the most intense event or action, for example "I am struggling against a wolf". Then I relate what happened just before and right after. The dream's description becomes substantially more vibrant when you see yourself at the very heart of the action. Furthermore, the significant emotional experience depicted in the dream might even instantly return.

As mentioned previously, dreams have the unfortunate tendency to slip away very quickly when one fails to jot them down upon waking up. Postponing writing down a dream is always risky. Whenever you awaken from an important dream in the middle of the night, write it down immediately to make sure it does not slip away. At the very least, make a list of all the words that will help recall the key images upon waking up. A good way is to keep a notebook or your Dream Journal with a reading light within easy reach, or a flashlight if someone else is around, to avoid sleep interruption. You could also keep a box of soft pastels or oil pastels at your fingertips in case you need to act quickly to make a sketch of a nightmare.

Important or Recurring Images

In any dream, please consider as important any image you find fascinating, intriguing or attractive, or images that turn you off … in short, anything that stirs up strong reactions. These images often, but not systematically, contain the essence of the dream's message. There have been a few times when I discovered the key meaning of a dream within a wisp of straw beside my house, after working all the images that had seemed important at first sight.

An important image that keeps coming back in your dreams is called a recurring image; the meaning might be the same every time, with minor differences. Some dreamers will have many dreams about the paternal home while others will recall a scene from a dream dating back several weeks or months ago. These images are particularly important for creating a personal dream dictionary, since they point out a series of dreams indicating a progressive deployment of the psyche.

Describing Recent Life Events

Taking note of life events gives access to the dream's context, a complex web of events and circumstances having symbolic connotations. The context often helps to grasp the dream's existential message, at the very moment when it is jotted down or later on when reading the contents again. For example, in one of my dreams, I saw a house constantly whipped up by gusts of wind, and I never seemed to be able to close the windows and to keep it in order. A pregnant woman was preparing her baby's trousseau, acting like everything was normal in the house, but there was also a young girl tearing everything apart and turning everything upside down.

On re-reading the dream one year after putting an end to a love relationship, I realised it was accurately reflecting my deepest feelings at the time; I was indeed in the throes of an emotional storm, torn between two parts of myself. While I pretended that I was doing fine and wanted a family life of my own, I kept making a mess and picking fights, knowing deep down inside my love relationship was not nurturing. How come I couldn't become aware of this when I had this dream, despite the evidence? I definitely had to resolve my inner conflict before acknowledging a house exposed to raging winds is not a safe place to live.

Jotting down recent life events on a piece of paper often makes it possible to understand instantly the relevance with the dream, though this quick interpretation could be misleading. Taking note of the context is the bare minimum required if you do not have either the time or the energy for dreamwork. Context provides crucial information which could help eventually understanding the dream.

Right Page of the Dream Journal: Decoding the Dream's Message

Elucidating the Dream's Message

The right page of the Dream Journal is used for elucidating the dream's message (see example at the end of this chapter). Discovering the message might be easier than you think; with a little bit of practice, you can all make it. No need to be an expert in dreams. On the contrary, only the dreamer ultimately holds the keys to understanding the meaning of his dreams.

On the right page of the Dream Journal, you write down the dream's number and title to make it easier to keep track of your dreams. Also specify the chosen dreamwork method, again to make it possible to spot this key information at a glance when reading or referring to your Dream Journal. Use preferably a Dream Journal with unlined paper, in case you want to draw or paint your dreams. If ever you need more space for illustrating a dream, use a large piece of paper, then take a picture of it, print it and glue it to the right page of your Journal.

There are lots of ways you can discover the dream's existential message. In this book, I am proposing the most simple and efficient methods as well as brief methods. With a little experience, you will come to identify your favorite ones and to decide which ones are suitable for every dream type. In some cases, elucidating the message requires using a number of dreamwork approaches for the same dream. Furthermore, it could be interesting to try many different methods for one same dream, just because each one of them might provide more depth to the message.

These methods have been broken down into three different chapters:

- The brief methods outlined in Chapter 3 are particularly useful when there is little time for dreamwork. These methods might help – but not systematically – to grasp momentarily the essential message of a dream, even if that means subsequently using more in-depth methods to provide additional nuance to the message. Other approaches get you directly involved in the dream. Considering they require a lower degree of emotional involvement than with experiential methods, they might help you feel safe, and could be more appropriate at times when you are feeling vulnerable.
- Experiential methods outlined in Chapter 4 teach how to explore dreams in-depth for the purpose of highlighting the existential message. They help to delve further into the "unknown self" and have a significant impact on an emotional level, which facilitates assimilation of the message. In some instances, a dream might remain a mystery, it could be that the time has not yet come to get the message, or the psyche is not ready to acknowledge it. Indeed, I have observed that people know how to protect themselves in the face of upsetting insights until they feel ready to face them; it is

therefore very important for that to be so. Our psyche has its own natural wisdom and our inner journey unfolds with the right timing at the right pace.

- Chapter 5 covers the most frequently used art-therapy dreamwork methods allowing to illustrate dreams through visual arts. These are extremely powerful methods to reconnect with the specific atmosphere of a dream, as well as to explore the dream, getting a feel of its effects, specifying its nature and grasping its emotional impact. Drawing or painting a dream scene further clarifies the message acutely. These methods do not require specific artistic skills; you just need to be willing to use lines, shapes, colors and a variety of media. You will find in Chapter 5 questionnaires and guidelines to use writing along with art creation, as well as recommendations about art materials.

Practical Applications

Once you understand the dream's message, you might see clearly the path to walk, the action to implement about a situation, the needed decision or the attitude that needs changing in your life. Your dream will inform you about an important aspect of your life experience, especially when using an experiential method for in-depth exploration.

In any event, if you understood the dream's existential message, it is important to quickly decide what tangible actions are required; otherwise, its meaning might fade from memory. If you get important information from the dream, make a decision about the actions to take and write them down on the right page of your Journal. The actions you take will be helpful to the extent that they are tangible, accurate and realistic, and take into account who you are, based on your tastes, preferences and limits. For example, you could simply do a ritual honoring the dream's meaning.

You can use these practical applications as a reminder; read them from time to time to see what remains to be done, what is no longer relevant and what has been accomplished.

Left Page of the Dream Journal

Date: _____ Dream #: _____

Dream type: _____

Existential message: _____

_____

_____

_____

Title: _____

Description *(dream story)*:

_____
_____
_____
_____
_____
_____
_____
_____
_____
_____
_____
_____

Important and/or recurring images:

_____
_____
_____
_____

Recent life events:

_____
_____
_____
_____
_____

Right Page of the Dream Journal

Title: _____Dream #: _____

Method(s) used for dreamwork: _____

Elucidation of the dream's message:

Practical applications or ritual to honor the dream's message:

_____

_____

_____

_____

How to Remember Dreams

- Set the alarm clock 15 to 20 minutes in advance to take time to recall the images and sensations upon waking. This is often effective enough to remember your dreams. Please avoid reviewing your daily schedule; you might want to stay in touch with the images and feelings present on waking, laying still in bed and keeping your eyes closed.
- After holding still for a while, try another position you like to sleep in. As a matter of fact, it is easier to remember a dream by getting into the position you were sleeping in.
- Keep a pencil and a notebook by the bed. When you wake up at night, jot down a few key words about your dream's images so that they can be brought back to your mind when you read them in the morning, given one often wakes up at night following a dream. You do not even need to turn on the light to write down these few words.
- Upon waking, please take note right away of the dreams you remember since the images will quickly vanish. Dreams will return to your mind in reverse order, the last scene in the last dream followed with the previous scene, then the second-last dream, and so on.
- Open your Dream Journal every morning, whether you had a dream or not. If you did not have any, please take note of the blurry sensations and emotions present upon waking up, and make up a night dream. It will include unconscious cues as though it was an actual dream, and dreamwork on these cues will be possible. In the face of the determination displayed, the unconscious will finally capitulate, and you will have dream material.
- Value all cues. At the end of the night, please note everything even if it is only a sound, an image or a sensation as if they were dreams, and your dreamwork will be profitable.
- The more you value your dreams and work with them, the more they return to your mind.
- Use the incubation approach. While falling asleep, affirm repeatedly that you will remember your dreams upon waking up in the morning.
- Initiate a dialogue about your resistance to remembering your dreams. You might ask questions like: "*Why are you staying away from me?*" and listen to the answers that will come naturally. As for me, I once had the following answer "*You have enough dream material to review for now, just work on the dreams you currently have.*" This answer was in fact consistent with my current reality. Once this dream material was finally elucidated, I was able to remember my dreams.

3
Creative Writing Methods for Dreamwork

In this chapter, ten different creative writing methods for dreamwork are presented. They all require little time and are particularly useful in circumstances where an in-depth approach is not preferred, for lack of time or energy.

Some of them will be all that is needed to quickly identify the dream's existential message, while others will provide for a few important clues about the dream's meaning without revealing the global existential message. Nevertheless, they will enhance self-consciousness, which is a very valuable result per se. Studies have demonstrated that the mere act of trying to make sense of one's dreams may have beneficial impacts. As an example, Pesant and Zadra (2010) mention clinical results where dreams recurring over months or years stopped after a single therapy session, even if their meaning had not been understood yet.

I recommend trying a number of these methods a few times, in order to find out your preferred approaches, the ones that work effectively for you. Over time, you will also be able to do dreamwork in a more flexible way, selecting the appropriate method for each dream type and tapping into a wide range of potential methods. With practice only will you ultimately find your own personal way to elucidate dreams.

Spontaneous Associations Methods

Two methods are offered, the first one requires taking note of spontaneous associations to dream images, and the second one is called the heuristic map.

Spontaneous Associations to Dream Images (Written Form)

The first method involves writing down any association coming spontaneously to mind when thinking about a dream. The following may be included in your spontaneous associations: your feelings and impressions upon waking up, your response to the dream and what goes through your mind upon writing it down, any objects, persons or situations that the dream images remind you of, as well as any instant assumption about the meaning of the dream. To help you find the relevant associations, you may focus on the specific images coming up when thinking about your dream. As a matter of fact, the message is often conveyed through images. In other words, the message can reveal itself if you pay attention to the images per se. Keep going back to a same dream image in order to find out about any associations coming to mind, then proceed with the other ones.

Just as importantly, keep in mind that spontaneous associations are not interpretations. There is a widely held misconception that feelings and ideas about a dream upon waking up are good enough to elucidate it. Frequently, it only reflects our defense mechanisms and our conscious mind. Often, more extensive dreamwork will push us into totally unforeseen directions; consequently, if we stick to spontaneous associations to try elucidating a dream, we might miss the substantive existential message.

So why should you take note of spontaneous associations? One of the purposes is to help you re-immerse into the dream's context the day you will undertake in-depth dreamwork. Moreover, this method has a way of clearing out of the way any associations on your mind, which makes you available for a more profound message. Therefore, it is interesting to write down any spontaneous associations even when you have time for in-depth work. Although the existential message is not necessarily revealed through spontaneous associations, they often show the way to understanding the dream's message.

Let's not forget that such associations may instantly highlight a dream's message and an inner certitude may arise from it; in that event, there is just no need for extensive dreamwork.

Application Example

The Planes

I see four planes up in the sky; there is a brown one on my right side, a white one on my left side and two small ones in front of me. I am the pilot in the brown plane. My hands are tight on the steering wheel (it's a car wheel), and it's vibrating. I am flying diagonally in front of the white plane and the small left plane.

Thinking to myself that I would have liked to pilot my husband's plane, I feel disappointed; then in my dream, I realise that my husband's plane is the brown one and it's the one I am piloting!

My spontaneous associations

First association: The day before, I went to see Always, a movie featuring airmen. This movie touched me deeply given my brother is a pilot.

Second association: I am currently aware that I am always unhappy with myself; I just can't appreciate my true worth. In my dream, I could have focused on piloting the plane, enjoying the ride, especially since the plane was the one that I was interested in. At first sight, the dream's message might be to acknowledge my own qualities and have more self-appreciation.

The first spontaneous association to this dream refers to the context of the movie; to some extent, it might turn out to be useful for understanding the dream's meaning, but it is meaningless in itself. Having seen a movie with similar images is not an adequate explanation of the fact I had such a dream. Any images we remember are personal and arise from the unconscious. In other words, the unconscious mind resonates with images seen in a movie and makes use of them.

The second spontaneous association is likely pretty consistent with the dream's existential message; however, it will remain an interesting assumption till completion of the dreamwork. This dream will also be addressed in Chapter 4, for the purpose of demonstrating the Gestalt identification method.

Spontaneous Associations to Dream Images (Graphic Form): The Heuristic Map

I recently learned about heuristic maps or mental charts called "Mind Maps" by Buzan and Buzan (2008). Jobin (2013, 2002) uses a similar tool called a mental map or "bubble diagram". While serving to collect our key ideas about a specific topic in a graphic form, heuristic maps are frequently used to facilitate learning.

Applying this graphic tool to dreamwork helps quickly visualise any important images and associations. Proceeding in two steps is useful: First, take note of all the associations related to the dream images that come to mind; second, organise this material to link overlapping ideas together through a series of bubbles and branches. Placed at the center of the map, the dream's title is highlighted with colors, tri-dimensional lettering and quick diagrams. Key images of the dream all radiate from the center.

The branches representing the spontaneous associations radiate from each element in the diagram. Make sure you will have enough space, using for example a large sheet (46 × 61 cm/18" × 24"), even if it means to take a picture of it and print it in a smaller size to insert into your Dream Journal subsequently.

Application Example

Applied to the previous dream about planes, the heuristic map looks as follows:

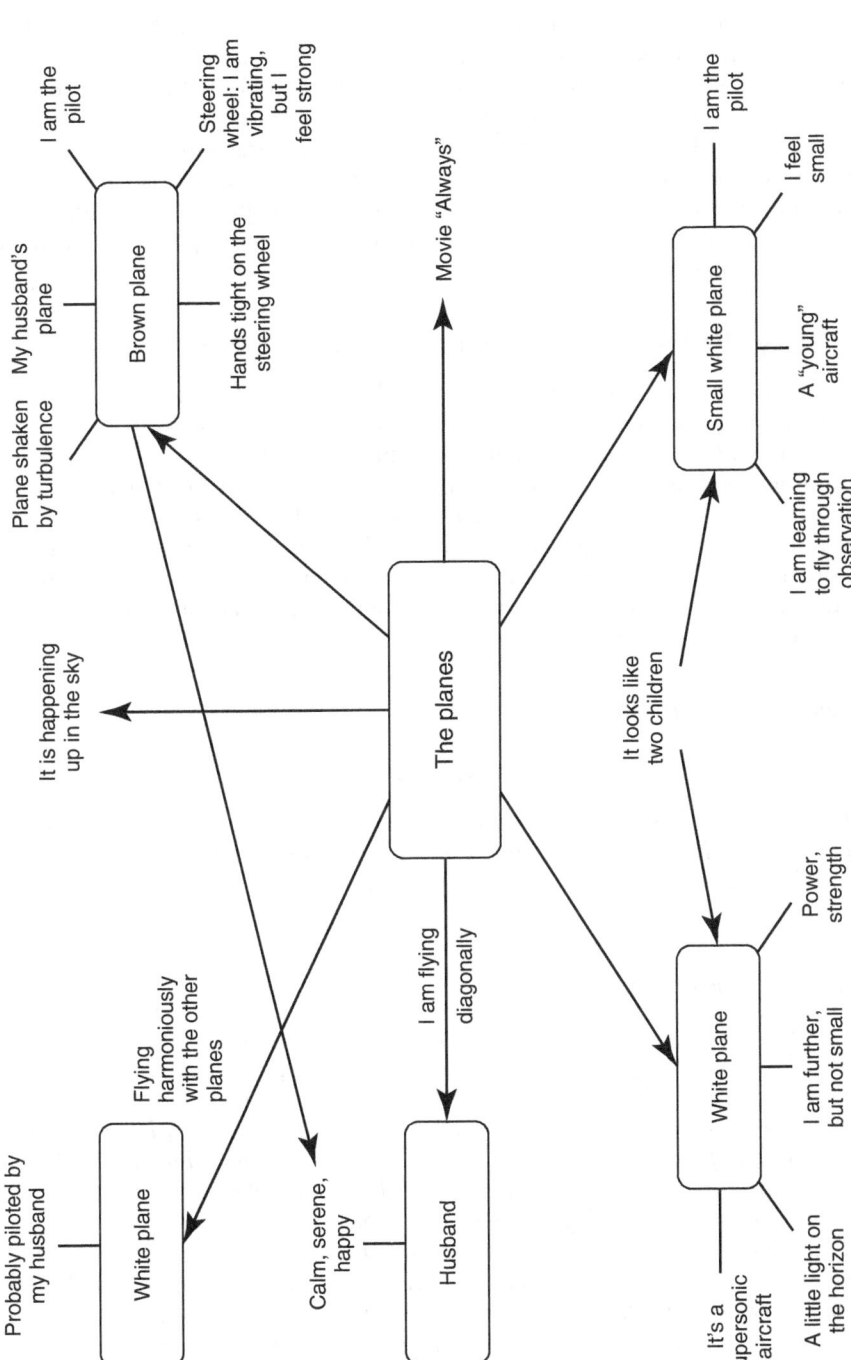

Figure 3.1 Heuristic Map for the Dream Titled "The planes".

Twenty-five years after the first edition of this book in French, I applied the heuristic map method to the above dream and a new association emerged. As a matter of fact, this dream dated back to 1990 when I only had one child. My daughter was born in 1993. Therefore, she was just *a little light on the horizon* in 1990! From hindsight, it seems this dream was foreseeing there would be another addition to the family, since I was effectively wondering if I felt like welcoming a second child and if I was strong enough for this. This dream was an affirmative answer in itself. Sometimes, dreaming precedes conscious thought, as Jung (2010) said.

Identifying the Key Feeling from a Dream

A very efficient and quick method, the following is often all that is needed to understand the existential message from a dream. It is inspired from the *Feeling Therapy* approach. Joseph Hart, Ph.D. and Richard Corrière, Ph.D., psychotherapists and Feeling Therapy practitioners, describe it in a very interesting book titled *Les maîtres-rêveurs* (2014 or *The Dream Makers*, 1979). The purpose of their approach is to highlight the predominant feelings of the dreamer. All you have to do thereafter is to ask yourself in what specific circumstances you have such feelings, with whom, at what time of the day and where. It is often extremely revealing!

Application Example

The Rose, My Center

In my dream, I am touching with my index finger a white rose with pink petals spread over a flat surface; I immediately feel « galvanised » by this touch. I know I have just touched my center.

Dreamer's comments

I accurately identify the predominant feeling in my dream, which is I feel "galvanised". This word is important, given it is clearly stated in the dream. The Feeling Therapy method is all the more relevant as my dream is focused on this particular feeling. Therefore, it is appropriate to ask myself where I feel as if I am galvanised in my waking life. I first take time to check how this term is defined in the dictionary. It means "to stimulate, to excite, to thrill". I marvel at how my dream uses terms whose precise meaning is beyond the reach of my conscious mind!

I specifically recognise the feeling from the dream. I am wondering what triggers such a feeling in my waking life. After some thought, I realise this is how I feel when I think of a specific project that I have been cooking up lately! Then I become aware that this project holds a huge potential to energise me, which is central, given I am literally "touching the center" of my being when thinking about it! It confirms this project is invaluable for me. This is an important piece of information, given I have been reluctant to undertake such an extensive project up to now. What I am getting from the dream is crucial, as my project is highly significant for me. This is the existential message I got from the dream, and my decision is being informed through it.

Meditating on an Elusive Sensation from a Dream

This method was adapted from the focusing technique developed by Eugene Gendlin (1998). Upon waking, what is left from a dream is frequently an elusive sensation, a feeling hard to identify because it is very fuzzy but whole at the same time. No image can be recalled and only a blurry feeling remains. The dream might also offer quite a mix of feelings and leave nothing else but a sense of unknown.

The above method involves taking as few minutes to stay connected with the elusive sensation, which means staying focused on it and feeling it to get a taste of it, without intellectualisation. As you keep focusing on it, you will notice that words describing its uniqueness are beginning to emerge. Please take note of these as they arise.

The elusive sensation might remain elusive. And it is quite normal, given the purpose of the exercise is to feel something still very vague but just beginning to emerge from the unconscious mind. Meditation is the most important step here, as focusing on the feeling will probably cause it to become more explicit in an upcoming dream.

However, the elusive sensation might also become clearer over the meditation process; whenever this happens, please just ask yourself to which sphere in your life the elusive sensation refers to, just like for the other approach previously outlined. Where and when did you feel something similar in your waking life? The answer to this question might lead to the dream's existential message.

Using this method might also be appropriate for dreams whose images and story are recalled upon waking up, but involve a similar vague and blurry sensation, just like in the following.

Application Example

The Clown's Train

I am with old co-workers in my college teaching years. I want to refurbish an old train no longer in use with their help. I am painting the outside of a train car using an array of beautiful colors and I am refurbishing the inside as a shelter for the use of my family. The other people do the same. Train cars are all connected; I am going for a site tour hand in hand with my co-workers. I am wearing a clown makeup and the other people too. The train is traveling and I am lying down with my family in my own train car. I realise I am sick and tired of being tossed around. Then as I remember where I am and our special common project, I do not mind being tossed and bounced along anymore.

Dreamer's comments

After writing down my dream, an elusive sensation persisted. Staying focused on the blurry sensation, I could only see a profusion of different colors at first, then I focused on the fuzzy feeling again. As the sensation was getting clearer, I became aware I had some sense of joy and well-being. This came from feeling connected to other people – just like the connected train wagons – and from being part of a community.

I came to realise the dream's meaning after getting in touch with my feelings in a clearer way. I am currently developing professional relationships with other art therapists, and the dream points out the sense of well-being coming from this. In addition, this existential message is confirmed by other features of the dream, given the characters are former co-workers, with whom I was entertaining a very satisfactory relationship as a group. On the other hand, the clown character has long been referring to my professional life, and symbolises for me the sacredness of my being's individuation through my career path. Therefore, here I am also using the spontaneous associations to the « clown » term to confirm the message from this dream, which is to go ahead with my private practice project in art therapy.

Taking Away a Part of a Dream

This method involves taking away some segments of a dream to consider whether any change would result from this. This brief approach was proposed by Jill Mellick (1996); she reviews the dream as if each important figure was no longer in it, asking herself what the impact of such an omission would be. She questions what would be missing or whether anything essential is brought by a figure. As a result, the theme of the dream and the existential message are highlighted.

Application Example

If this approach was applied to the previous dream about the clown's train, the result would be as follows:

If This Was Taken Away	This Would Be Missing
My former co-workers from college	A positive sense of belonging
An old abandoned train	Something abandoned will be reused
An array of beautiful colors	Joy and art
My family	A sense of intimacy and belonging

If This Was Taken Away	This Would Be Missing
Train cars all connected	A sense of connection
The site tour	Creating a community circle
The clown	The Self
The traveling train	A sense of progression
Lying down with my family in my train car	A sense of inhabiting my own world
Being bounced along	Encountering bumps and unpleasant surprises
Accepting to be bounced along	Refusing to be bounced along would result in giving up a project possibly challenging but bringing a sense of belonging.

Here also, the above approach enabled me to get a support message about a full-time private practice I had just initiated at that time. The dream also stresses the joy of developing professional relationships with art therapy colleagues through my work. I had reached the same conclusion using the meditation approach, which shows that the existential message can be identified through various methods. It often is a matter of personal preference for one approach or another. When one does not work for you, just try another one.

Changing the Ending of a Dream

This approach is inspired from Carl Jung; he sometimes asked his clients to use active imagination to continue the dream story where it stopped. For most dreams, there is no specific ending. Writing a more gratifying ending in your Dream Journal generates an inner sense of competency and gives the psyche the message to develop new skills. For example, if you act in a dream so as to experience something fulfilling or to feel your own power, this will subsequently transfer into your waking life. The dream serves as a laboratory where you get a feel of success, helping you become more successful in waking life!

Application Example

Following the dream titled "*The rose, my center*" (see p. 48), I had the following dream:

The Secret Meeting

I am meeting with four or five persons. I am sitting among them and they entrust me with some kind of mission or spiritual role that stirs a reaction of fear in me. I do not understand what the mission is and I am reluctant to say yes. I can't remember if they received an answer from me.

Dreamer's comments

Upon waking up, I decide to change the ending of this dream and to write it down: I don't know what this mission is, but I think it reflects exactly what I want to accomplish in life. So, my answer is an enthusiastic "yes", despite the fact I am feeling afraid.

This dream being a follow-up to the one titled "The rose, my center", which brought me to understand a specific project was arising from the center of my being, I realise it is about the same issue, meaning I am invited to move ahead with my own spiritual journey through this project.

Rewriting a Dream

Kaplan Williams (1987), a Jungian analyst and founding director of the Senoï Jungian Institute in Berkeley, California, recommends rewriting any parts of a dream you are not happy with, especially the incomplete ones.

You can change your attitude towards a situation, insist on sentiments poorly expressed, change your behavior; in other words, you can change anything you are unhappy with concerning your behavior or the dream's outcomes. It is a matter of creating an inner sense of satisfaction and a profound sense that an issue has been resolved. Even if you do not necessarily understand the many forces at play, the resolving will have an impact on your psyche. It is as if your psyche starts embracing the new programming you are sliding into. This approach is a very efficient personal transformation process, especially if applied to many dreams and for some time.

Rewriting a dream sometimes is all that is needed to find the dream's existential message, because of the contrast between the dream's content and what you would have ideally liked experiencing in it.

This technique might have another interesting impact, that is to pave the way for lucid dreaming since it teaches how to take action consciously on your dreams. When you rewrite dreams, you effectively take action into the dreamworld.

Application Example

A 40-year-old woman had the following dream.

A Liberating Nightmare

Before leaving home, I take time to check whether the door is locked. It is not. I am surprised about this and I open the door for a second check. I see a man dressed up as a paper boy; he is wearing a navy cap and is slightly crouched down below the mailbox. He reaches out to catch me with his hand. This man has my father's face. Since I am afraid, I start whining to get assistance from people around me. Then I literally start screaming. Then my husband wakes me up.

Dreamer's comments

I made the decision to change this dream upon my waking up. Instead of letting the man catch me, I fought back and caught him. I saw myself punching him and using a judo move. It did not work. Then I repeatedly visualised these images in my mind and finally replayed the scene added with the screaming; I saw myself doing a judo move, knocking and tackling the man to the ground with my foot as if I were taming a wild beast, then I shouted a victory cry as would Tarzan … Then my breathing changed instantly. Deep belly breathing just happened organically for several minutes. Powerlessness, fear, inhibition of action had been transformed into fighting and victory.

This woman felt that her dreamwork was a turning point in her personal growth process. From that moment on, she felt as though, in her own words, the jailer "had taken a bit of a hit"! The morning after, she woke up feeling more joyful, having more energy and less muscular tension.

Programming Changes in Recurring Dreams

As mentioned in Chapter 1, recurring dreams are dreams that keep coming back at more or less regular intervals. A desired change can be programmed with this type of dream. This technique aims to accustom the psyche to engage in more rewarding behaviors in dreams. It is inspired by the methods of the Senoï people from Malaysia who developed a complex system of intervention into their dreams. The goal of the process is always to head for positive results (Garfield, 1983).

First, it is important to clearly identify your intention and then formulate it in a short sentence describing the expected result. This technique specifically applies to recurrent dreams in which the same situation is re-experienced over and over again. It is about repeating the change one wishes to make, by reiterating a phrase in a state of relaxation, just before going to sleep, for example "I am dreaming that I successfully break free from the paralyzing force". It can also be repeated several times a day, to take it in. It is important to persevere, as it can take several weeks or months to change recurrent dreams.

Application Example

I was told by a close relative that she often loses her purse or her way in her dreams and then she feels anxious because she never receives help from anybody. I suggested that she fall asleep every night thinking that there will be someone to help if she has that dream again.

After a few months, she told me that programming her dreams had successfully reassured her and that her dreams had been less dreadful over the last while. In her dream life, as in her waking life, she was feeling less and less helpless.

Programming Incubation Dreams

Programming an incubation dream means providing yourself with the conditions required to have the night dreams you want to have. Garfield (1995/1983) mentioned there was a similar tradition in ancient Greece where the Pilgrims visited Asclepius's temple, the God of medicine, in order to have healing dreams. The Pilgrims effectively had healing dreams, probably because of the fulfillment of a number of psychological favorable conditions.

This method requires to first decide on the dream you want to experience: A healing dream, one providing a solution to a problem you are unable to resolve, a creative dream about your next painting, the next book to write, a project to undertake, etc. It can be a lucid dream, a telepathic one or a clairvoyant one, etc. Possibilities are endless. The difference between this method and the previous one is subtle: This time you are programming a dream type and in the previous one, you were programming a change in the psyche.

State your intention in a short sentence, for example "I will dream that I am flying", "I will dream that I am doing a painting". Say this sentence repeatedly at bedtime or throughout the day, as for the previous method. Once again, perseverance is important.

Patricia Garfield (1983) pointed out the psychological conditions that can help program a dream: To have a clear and precise intention rather than a vague one; to repeat the intention at bedtime, in a relaxation or sleep-like state; to engage in activities related to the dream project during the day or before going to bed, for example reading on the subject. She also specified that creating immersive conditions increases the chances to have the night dream you want, for example doing activities related to the project for two or three days, or more if possible, in a space where nothing will come to distract you.

You can also have an incubation dream in less favorable conditions. If you are deeply concerned about a problem that you have tried to solve to no avail, you are more likely to get an answer if you ask for a solution to come from your night dreams.

Application Example

During my specialised training in art therapy in California, I had the chance to do an internship in an institution for pre-teens struggling with emotional disorders. I had a hard time acting with the right attitude, and sometimes I was very dissatisfied with my work with them. As a last resort, I asked for answers from my night dreams, to understand where the problem was. Then I had this dream:

The Car with No Brakes

I am sitting in a big American car, in the passenger seat. One of the children I am treating at that institution is driving the car that has no brakes.

Dreamer's comments

Upon waking, the meaning of the dream became clear to me: The issue experienced by these troubled children is often that they need boundaries (they have no "brakes"). By letting the child drive, I was not setting enough boundaries. My Rogerian[1] humanist conception of non-intervention in the client's process could not apply to this particular clientele. So, I revised my attitude from this new perspective and I immediately noticed positive impacts. I was using night dreaming this way for the first time and I was pretty astounded at the incredibly fair and accurate response I got.

Exploring Dream Symbols

Symbols are the language of the unconscious mind arising spontaneously in night dreams, art, active imagination, sandplay therapy,[2] mental imagery or visions. Symbols play a dynamic role; when they are activated, they have the power to advance the psyche toward its realisation (Stein, 2009). They organise and structure the psychic energy: They pick it up, contain it and guide it. Through them, content that is still completely unconscious is trying to make its way to the conscious mind. Conscious work with symbols makes them more effective, as in dreamwork.

Carl Jung is one of the first and most important psychiatrists to have explored symbols in dreams, artwork and imagination (Jung, 1993/1953, 1964; Johnson, 1986). He developed working methods that make it possible to effectively explore the meaning of symbols; among them, there is the amplification approach.

---

1 Inspired by Carl Rogers (1961), this approach is client-oriented. It means the therapist's interventions are not oriented towards pre-determined therapeutic goals but is based on the client's experience during therapy sessions.

2 Sandplay therapy is a psychotherapeutic approach where the client is invited to create an imaginary scenario in a wood box filled with sand, using various miniature figures. (Weinrib, 2004; Kalff, 1973).

Dictionary of Symbols

The amplification of symbols, by means of dictionaries of symbols for example, develops and enriches the unconscious content of images, thus adding a supra-personal dimension, since it is found in many individuals and many cultures, creating a sense of belonging to the human community (Lévesque, 2015).

A dictionary of symbols, as a method to elucidate the meaning of dream content, involves collecting information about a symbol from collective data such as myths, fairy tales, religious traditions, archaeological data or others. According to Johnson (2009/1986), Jung was very surprised to find in his patients' dreams the occurrence of very old images and symbols, sometimes even belonging to cultures that the dreamer could not know of.

Using a dictionary of symbols is particularly useful when archetypal images arise in a dream, for example a known universal symbol commonly found in our culture or even in many traditions, or in tales, mythology or legends. A few examples are a cross, a mandala,[3] a circle, a square, a snake, a rose, colors, numbers, well-known figures, etc. Even then, the most effective way to use a dictionary of symbols is to exercise critical thinking; when reading the different meanings of a symbol, the possible avenues to be considered are the ones that seem to mean something to you. In other words, you should avoid putting ready-made meanings on images from your dreams. That is in fact why I recommend using dictionaries of symbols, rather than dictionaries of dreams which are found in large numbers on the market, since the former generally offer far more potential meanings than the latter.

Many books about dreams only suggest using dictionaries of dreams. In my opinion, it is at best a short method, generally inadequate. The images and symbols in night dreams are personal. Their meaning differs from person to person; it can also change in the same individual, according to his particular situation. That is why the idea of making one's own dictionary of dreams is of great interest.

Application Example

The following dream, *Zeus' finger*, was described in the first chapter, in the series about snakes; it clearly illustrates the insights dictionaries of symbols can bring about on what is going on. Here it is:

Zeus' Finger

Like the one in Michelangelo's painting, Zeus throws a lightning bolt with his finger and it penetrates my third eye. At that moment, the word **empowerment** *comes to my mind.*

---

3 In Sanskrit, the word "Mandala" means magic circle; it is a circle with a centre divided into four sections or into multiples of four. See Jung, 1972.

Comments

Zeus, Michelangelo and the third eye are universal symbols. The arising of the Zeus symbol in the dream comes as a surprise. It is such a universal symbol, totally out of the dreamer's daily life, that there is good reason to wonder who exactly Zeus was, how the Greeks perceived him and what he symbolised. It is one way to gather more information about the dream itself. Now, among the many meanings associated to Zeus and the third eye in the dictionary of symbols by Gheerbrant and Chevalier (1998), here are the ones that spoke to my client:

- Zeus: When he throws a lightning bolt (which happens in the dream), Zeus, father of the gods and humans, symbolises spirit and the enlightenment of human intelligence, illumination and intuition from the Divine; he is the source of truth (p. 1036).
- Third eye: It is the organ of the inner vision; therefore, this is an external expression of the heart's eye; inner vision unifies love and intellect (p. 686).

The above meanings confirm that the dreamer has a growing sense of power over her emotions and her needs; she can now respond better and feels less overwhelmed by her emotions. She also knows they are related to her relationship with her father that she is currently exploring in-depth. She feels a better integration between her intellect and her emotions, which is confirmed by the dream's symbols. Her self-knowledge and her dreams undoubtedly facilitate the use of the dictionary in a way that truly applies to her situation. The more you know yourself, the more you can effectively use dictionaries of symbols.

Now, all you have to do is to try all the brief methods. Please use them regularly and experiment with them. You will find out the ones that work best for you and that suit you personally.

4

Experiential Dreamwork Methods

The five experiential methods presented in this chapter form the basis of almost all the dreamwork techniques presented in this book and their variants. Although quite different from a technical perspective, the methods based on graphical representation of dreams described in Chapter 5 are also based on the Gestalt and Jungian methods outlined below.

These methods thus help to penetrate the symbolic universe of dreaming and to explore it. Essentially, they enable to relive a dream and to re-enter into the emotional realm aroused by images and situations. Understanding a dream is not an intellectual process, it essentially is an affective process. Consciously reliving emotions provides insight into what it is all about: the primordial existential message, often urgent, that a dreamer delivers to himself through a dream. Ultimately, only the dreamer is capable of interpreting his dreams. Indeed, the final criterion of a successful interpretation is the certainty brought to the dreamer, a certainty that leaves no room for doubt.

The methods proposed in this book allow in-depth work on oneself. As such, they stand out from the brief methods, which remain superficial and require less emotional commitment from the dreamer. Experiential methods initiate a profound process of change; in this sense, they require a greater commitment of time and effort. This is why some people only use them occasionally while others keep them for their most important dreams or use them regularly. It is up to individuals to choose for themselves on the basis of the situation and their personality.

The last step of these methods is to highlight the existential message. While I systematically dedicate a few lines on how to achieve this step, the basic information on the existential message is detailed in Chapter 2. Referring frequently to it may be helpful at the beginning.

Identification with Dream Figures

Identification is truly the basis of any Gestalt dreamwork; it is also my favorite method, with the Jungian dialogue process, besides the artwork approaches.

The Gestalt perspective considers that a dream is an existential message, which means a message delivered through the unconscious mind about the dreamer's life (Perls, 1992). Is it close enough to the *breakthrough dreaming* approach of *Les Maîtres-Rêveurs* (*The Dream Makers*, 1977; see Corrière and Hart, 2014). A breakthrough dream refers to your unconscious mind breaking through your conscious mind, which disrupts the status quo in your person-ality. While dreams are not all significant breakthrough dreams, they are all messengers of the unconscious mind.

From the Gestalt perspective, all elements from a dream (i.e. figures, objects, animals, monsters, details of the environment), in short everything in a dream, represent a part of yourself. I think this is the key to elucidating dream mes-sages. Once you consider your dreams in this way, you begin to understand what it is about: dreams totally and completely speak about yourself; they illustrate states of mind felt in your unconscious mind; they reflect precisely your conscious and unconscious experience. The hardest part is to understand that dreams, although symbolic, accurately portray what is going on in your inner world.

Here is how the process unfolds according to the Gestalt theory: first a part of oneself is alienated then projected on some element of a dream. For all kinds of conscious and unconscious reasons, we deny certain parts of our life experi-ence, perceived as shameful. To be spared from deep anxiety, which might arise if we perceived these "flaws" in ourselves, all kinds of defense mechanisms are used to alienate these emotions, feelings, desires and likes; in short, they are rejected from our experience and treated as if they did not exist.

Unfortunately, it is not that simple. Life experiences do not just vanish. In waking life, they are often projected on the people around us, that is to say attributed to others. For example, "I am not the one who is angry, it is the other one that is". In the dream world, this alienated life experience is projected on the dream's images; our experience is shown in images, but in symbolic forms because the unconscious mind considers the fact that we do not recognise them as belonging to us; therefore, life experience appears in the form of characters, known or not, animals, monsters, and even objects, interacting with each other. The relationships between different elements of a dream represent the way these parts interact in us.

These alienated aspects of our personality are important personal resources from which we are cut off. Nightmares are perfect examples. They reflect our fears; they often arise when we are confronted with difficult existential prob-lems and forced to call upon all our resources, feeling more or less overwhelmed with the events. They are among the most important dream experiences, because they precisely reveal those alienated parts and the missing resources.

In a typical nightmare, we are chased by someone or something: a monster, a thief, a threatening individual, etc. Actually, the hunter is simply the image of a part of us that is rejected, which is pursuing us. Indeed, everything we reject might eventually work against us until we restore a place for it inside of us. In addition, when we are having a nightmare, we only need to stop running away and to face the monster for it to stop being threatening. This drastic form was used with the sole aim of drawing our attention; once that goal is achieved, it is no longer necessary.

As an example, I dream about an alien and wake up freaked out over that image. Rereading the dream story is enough for me to re-experience a sense of fear. This image is self-explanatory; it is about an unknown part of me (an alien); the rest of the dream indicates it is associated with sexuality. However, no matter how hard I work on the image, its meaning remains elusive, probably because that part of me is such a huge unknown that I am just unable to identify it. Monitoring the progress of this image in my future dreams will be required to be able to figure out eventually what it represents. Based on the usual way dreams progress, the alien image will return, becoming ever clearer. And I will eventually access this unknown part of me.

The Gestalt method for identifying with a dream's elements enables us to take responsibility for these parts of ourselves in order to become more complete and in full command of our resources, with greater self-awareness. It requires reconnecting with the rejected life experience by identifying with the elements of a dream, which is the exact opposite of alienation or dis-identification.

Description of the Method

Step #1: Making a list of a dream's elements
Step #2: Identifying with the elements from the dream
Step #3: Identifying the existential message

Step #1: Making a List of a Dream's Elements

First, write down any image contained in the dream, i.e. characters, animals, monsters, objects, landscape features or decor elements. You can also add abstract elements: situations, actions, feelings, colors and numbers. These are all important because dream images contain all of the critical information.

Step #2: Identifying with the Elements from the Dream

This step involves taking the elements of the list one by one and identifying with them, starting with those that seem the most important, the lesser-known and the fascinating or significant ones.

"Identify with" involves using the "I" and the present tense, describing oneself as the character, the animal or the object, and writing down what spontaneously comes to mind by identifying with any character or object as depicted in the dream. For example, let's say that I am dreaming about a plane: "I am a plane flying in the sky ..." Now, "identifying with" means to become this character or this object for a moment, and to put oneself in its shoes.

It is very important to identify with only one element of the dream at a time. When nothing else comes up spontaneously or you feel a connection is made with your life experience, move on to another element of the dream. After a few ones, you will see the relationship between your dream and your waking life; a new light will be shed on a part of your life experience until then unclear. Step #3 of the identification method will be the next one.

Step #3: Identifying the Existential Message

The message from the dream reveals itself when you feel a connection between the dream images and the emotions experienced in your waking life. At the time when you write down the words that describe you as this or that element of the dream, an unexpected connection is instantaneously established between a dream and daily life.

After highlighting the passages from your writings that relate to aspects of your life experience (as shown in the following example), you will be able to identify the existential message providing you trust your feelings; the identified connections between the written passages and your waking life will contain the dream's message.

Application Example

The Planes

I see four planes up in the sky; there is a brown one on my right side, a white one on my left side and two small ones in front of me. I am the pilot in the brown plane. My hands are tight on the steering wheel (it's a car wheel), and it's vibrating. I am flying diagonally in front of the white plane and the left plane.

Realising I would have liked to pilot my husband's plane, I feel disappointed; then in my dream, I realise that my husband's plane is the brown one and it's the one I am piloting!

Step #1: Making a List of a Dream's Elements

- The brown plane;
- The white plane;
- The little plane on the right side, in front of me;
- The little plane on the left side, in front of me;
- The vibrating steering wheel;

- My husband (despite being only mentioned once, he is still part of my dream);
- The sky.

Step #2: Identifying with the Elements from the Dream

I am a brown plane. The pilot is Johanne; my steering wheel is vibrating a lot, which makes the pilot afraid; I do not know why I am brown. I am vibrating a lot … I feel I need strength to control myself and stay on track; that probably means I will encounter clouds, turbulences or air pockets along the way; I know I am in no danger of falling apart or breaking into pieces, although I am moving around a lot these days.

I am a white plane. I am presently flying high up in the sky; I do not know who is the pilot but I am flying; I seem to be flying together with the brown plane and the two smaller ones in front of me that are white as well. I think, in theory, that I am Johanne's plane, but right now Johanne is piloting the brown plane. I am flying in harmony and smoothly, together with the other ones.

I am a small white plane. I am flying with my mother-plane and my father-plane (this arose spontaneously inside of me when identifying with one of the two smaller planes). I know where I belong in this formation flight and I maintain my position. It makes me feel good. Although I feel small, I know how to fly; I seem to be my own pilot. I am a young plane; I am learning to fly by observing my parental planes.

I am the other small white plane (the left one). In fact, I am not small, I am just farther away. Right now, I am just a tiny point in space, I am traveling close to the speed of light; I am actually a supersonic aircraft, a very powerful aircraft. And I too am my own pilot. I am very powerful and very strong, but at this point I am just a small ray of light on the horizon.

I am the steering wheel that is vibrating a lot. I act as a guide; I have a circular configuration and I am divided in four. I am moving around a lot. In fact, I feel like I am shaking and that I am in danger of being ripped from the plane, but I know I am strong.

I am Johanne's husband. I am not part of the dream, but I have a plane that seems to be envied. I feel calm, serene and happy.

Step #3: Identifying the Existential Message

When I had this dream, I was going through a lot of emotional turbulence in the summer, bursting into tears without knowing why. Now, it took two months to figure out the reasons for these emotional roller coasters. I realised that a big change was taking place inside of me. This change would create greater serenity, a feeling that I envied my husband. Identifying with the elements of my dream allowed me to become aware of the following feelings:

Despite the emotional turbulences, I was feeling some serenity, even if I did not actually recognise it: The white plane flying in harmony and smoothly was a part of me. In addition, the dream ended with the realisation that I was in fact piloting my husband's plane. I need to recognise what I already have and appreciate it.

"I am in no danger of falling apart or breaking into pieces, although I am moving around a lot these days." The emotional turbulences I was going through were not dangerous and I was not at risk of breaking into pieces. Therefore, there was no need to be afraid of what was going on inside of me. I felt comforted by this aspect of the dream.

"I am strong." My basic structure was depicted by the steering wheel, which indeed represented a mandala: A circle divided into four sections. For me, this symbolised personal integrity. The steering wheel knew it was solid, despite everything. Here again, the dream indicated that my inner structure remained strong despite the current turmoil.

Finally, the dream advised me on the change that was taking place, thanks to two small planes. "I am a young plane and I am my own pilot" told me that something new was born and that it pointed toward greater autonomy. I also realised that even if it was still a small ray of light on the horizon, something very powerful was coming forward.

Six weeks after, this dream became crystal clear: Through this process I did not understand at first, I reconnected with a deeper layer of my being where deep sorrow was lurking, and I could quiet down a lot. It was the first time I was exploring this dream and it remained somewhat mysterious; however, I actually felt reassured about what was happening. It helped me tolerate that process I did not understand and allow it to unfold.

The existential message from this dreamwork was the following: *"Do not be afraid; you are going through gusty conditions right now, but it is not dangerous; something new and beautiful wants to be born in you."*

This existential message was not a self-imposed logical deduction; it felt profoundly true. That is why it had value and effect and I felt deeply reassured.

Gestalt Dialogue with Dream Figures

This method is somehow a variation of the previous one. It can be used alone, but for beginners, it is easier to use after dreamwork through the identification method. The technique involves identifying oneself alternately with two elements of the dream that are interacting. It allows to work on inner conflicts, what Perls (1972) called *polarities*. It sometimes completes the identification method.

The term *polarity* is defined as a conflict between two parts of oneself on opposite sides of the spectrum. Our behaviors or choices then range from one extreme to the other, creating within us an unending cycle with no way out or a continued state of indecision in relation to a specific situation, or else a feeling of always facing the same problem. Such a conflict usually leaves us with a bad feeling of hopelessness, the feeling of being unable to change whatever we do.

In fact, our energy is torn between two powerful forces that share the power, creating a state of tension and inner paralysis. Most of the time we resolve this intolerable situation by giving in first to one then to the other side.

In order to break free from their grip, we need to overcome the conflict by creating a new way of being that aligns the forces involved, making equal space for both polarities. Instead of running around in circles, we will then leverage the energy released by the resolution of the conflict. This energy now becomes available to deal with another polarity. Addressing one's polarities is an important issue of personal growth. The more you bring solutions to your inner conflicts, the more you increase the energy available within you and the more you head toward harmony, in other words toward serenity and inner peace.

Description of the Method

Step #1: Focusing on two interacting elements of the dream
Step #2: Writing down a dialogue between the two parties
Step #3: Identifying the state of conflict
Step #4: Initiating a resolution process
Step #5: Identifying the existential message

Step #1: Focusing on Two Interacting Elements of the Dream

First, it is a matter of identifying two opposing elements that interact in the dream or that, on the contrary, avoid each other, or two characters or two beings whose feelings, behaviors and attitudes are totally opposite or who are in outright conflict in the dream. The method is all the more relevant when applied to clearly conflicting parts of the dream.

Step #2: Writing Down a Dialogue Between the Two Parties

This step involves listening to what the two parties want to say to each other, writing it down. To do this, you must first identify with one of the characters or objects from the dream, then with the other party, who answers the first one, and so on. It is helpful to use two different color pencils, one for each party; or even to write with the dominant hand for one of the two parties and with the non-dominant hand for the other.

As an example, let's take a dream featuring an enthusiastic soldier and a serene young woman. You will first identify with one of the characters, in accordance with the identification method. As this young woman, you will tell the soldier what spontaneously comes to mind: *"I really feel I am the total opposite of you. I am serene, calm, determined and happy! You are always away, always on the move and you never settle down. I would not like to live like this!"* Then you will act like the soldier and respond to your interlocutor identifying with the soldier as best as you can, this way: *"I need action and stimulation and I need to be on the move and feel alive!"*

The dialogue will go on like this for a number of lines; you can even step out of the dream's environment while keeping on drawing inspiration from it. Just let any spontaneous reactions emerge as the young woman and then as the soldier, whether these reactions are part of the dream or not.

This preliminary dialogue ends when the two characters have shared what they think of each other (how different they are, the perception they have of each other, etc.), as well as their emotional response to one another. Then it will be time to move on to the next step.

Step #3: Identifying the State of Conflict

At this point, the conflict usually has become apparent through the dialogue. The more you emotionally respond to the other character, as felt and without censoring anything, the more the conflict is reflected in all its breadth through the dialogue. To ensure that the conflict is resolved, it is very important to first let the conflict unfold completely. I noticed that any inner conflict resolution follows a six-step process which basically unfolds spontaneously in the following order.

1 Confluence

What the dialogue is about
The conflict has not yet become apparent, since every party has not yet articulated the "vital message" that will differentiate it from the other.

What the dreamer is experiencing
The dreamer fails to clearly acknowledge which parts of himself are involved; he might even be confusing one with the other.

2 Polarisation

What the dialogue is about
The two parties are clearly identified and distinct from one another; the polarity is clear since both parties articulated their vital message.

What the dreamer is experiencing
The dreamer is able to identify what very real inner aspect of himself each party is associated to. He recognises two contradictory values that are often conflicted in him.

3 Opposition

What the dialogue is about
The two parties refuse to accept one another; one of them has to be eliminated; it is a fight to the death. The conflict is considered to be unsolvable.

What the dreamer is experiencing
The dreamer is often struggling with these same inner conflicts and feels helpless to resolve the conflict which usually is a long-standing one.

4 Deadlock

What the dialogue is about
The two parties become aware that no one is going to win, given that they are even forces so they will eventually accept the necessity of negotiating.

What the dreamer is experiencing
The dreamer becomes aware that the two forces are even and accepts that none of them will disappear, and subsequently considers a new possibility, to accommodate both parties instead of trying to eliminate one of them, which is impossible.

5 Negotiation

What the dialogue is about
The two parties are willing to accept one another, subject to certain conditions; they must be respectful of each other's most crucial values.

What the dreamer is experiencing
The dreamer anticipates that there are valuable aspects in each of the conflicted parties in him, even from the point of view of the opposite party; he does not feel as closed to the other party as before when identifying with it.

6 Resolution

What the dialogue is about
The conflict is resolved: Both parties make an agreement.

What the dreamer is experiencing
The parties feel that the agreement they made is real and is not a forced compromise, which would then be superficial and worthless, because it would not last long. Inner balance has just been achieved.

Step #3 thus involves checking where the conflict is at. It can be at any of the six stages mentioned above. It can even be resolved at stage #2. The simple fact of recognising through the dialogue that the other party exists might be enough to resolve the conflict. Listening to what both sides have to say may help us realise that we need both opposite parties in us. However, it is rarely that simple. The most unconscious parts in us are represented in the form of more negative images, that is to say, perceived as such. Most of the time, one of the two characters or objects represents a less tolerated and less recognised part of us. Much work needs to be done, step by step and painfully, for the purpose of integrating this part of us perceived as less positive.

In the above dialogue, I see the emergence of a polarity: The stable self and the unstable self. The latter is perceived in negative terms since it is personified by a soldier, which is a function I have a hard time valuing. Yet, the dialogue allows me to realise that I need these two types of energy; I need calm, serenity, the female quiet strength of character, as much as the energy personified by the soldier in order to be able to fight in real life, to face challenges, to go on my journey, in other words to be on the move. These two parties coexist inside of me and both seek to dictate different choices.

The opposition stage (Step #3) becomes clear further in the dialogue, as none of the two parties finds the other interesting or acceptable.

> Woman: Soldier, I think you are ugly, rough, primitive, aggressive and unstable.
>
> Soldier: I think for myself that you are indolent and you drag your feet when it comes to moving around!

Step #4: Initiating a Resolution Process

Identifying at what stage you are will help you know what step should be worked on to eventually resolve the conflict. You must willingly resume dialogue by simply asking your two sub-personalities to continue until an agreement is reached. An effective way of doing this would be to write down what both like about each other. In this particular instance, the deadlock step is the next. Further in the dialogue, you may notice how the female party reaches the point where it has no choice to take into consideration the other party, the soldier.

> Woman: I am reluctant to partner with you, because I really don't want to be like you. However, I could take advantage of your capacity to be on the move.
>
> Soldier: For myself, I do not want to be "indolent" like you, but I appreciate your emotional stability, your calm and your maturity; on the other hand, I do not want to let go of excitement.
>
> Woman: I am not interested in the excitement aspect. It feels like I cannot be who I am if I take this from you; I am not willing to lose my serenity.
>
> Soldier: You have no choice anyway, since you stop being calm whenever I show up. (Reference to the deadlock: You cannot pretend I'm not even here, because then I'm bothering you!)
>
> Woman: Yes, that is very true!

We are talking only about *initiating* the conflict resolution process since resolving it through a single dialogue is often impossible. What matters is that the dreamer sees where the problem is at and gives the dialogue a chance to be pursued. When not fully resolved, a conflict will reoccur in a new dream, in a similar form or with completely different symbols that will better reflect its new state, giving the dreamer a new opportunity to go even further with the dialogue. For example, if you find that the conflict is at the confluence stage, the most important thing to do is to treat the two parties as clearly distinct to enable a clear differentiation and assertion of their values and needs, which then allows to proceed with the polarisation step. Until that differentiation is made, little can be done. If the dialogue leads to differentiation, you will likely feel that your inner work is enough for the time being. Avoid continuing in such a case.

The successful differentiation at the polarisation stage implies that the vital message of both parties has been clearly asserted. You are in a state of confluence when feeling ambivalent about something (both *wanting something* and *not wanting it*). By looking more closely, you will be able to differentiate the two forces involved in the polarity and to understand that, although they are opposing ones, both represent values you hold important. The priority is to get both parties to state their vital message.

Similarly, if you find that a dialogue is at the opposition stage, then the most important thing is to simply acknowledge and accept that the two parties adamantly refuse to recognise each other as valuable. Temporarily accepting this as a fact without trying to change it is the wisest decision. In any case, any attempt at reconciliation would be useless.

Step #5: Identifying the Existential Message

I did not go on with the dialogue between the two parties and later realised that the conflict re-emerged in new dreams, in different forms. In the dialogue presented below, the theme about the capacity *to be on the move* reoccurs with new images and characters (see the dream about *The Angel and the Cripple* below). After working on several dreams featuring this theme, I finally resolved the conflict successfully. At this point, the most valuable thing I could do was to specifically state the conflict I was experiencing. It is important to avoid *forcing* resolution, because then it would not be lasting.

In the previous dialogue, it appears that serenity is a vital value for me, but being on the move, which means to continue to grow as an individual, is just as important. As long as the conflict was not resolved and I failed to achieve serenity and movement at the same time, these two forces caused interior division. I realised that the conflict had been resolved when I was able to leave behind a secure permanent job, with relative serenity, and to start the journey to private practice.

As I mentioned, it is important to identify at what stage the conflict is. If you find that you are in one of the first two stages, moving to the resolution stage in one try is very unlikely. Inner work through dialoguing is exhausting and real; we need time to change.

Application Example

The following is an excerpt from a polarity dream.

The Angel and the Cripple

I am looking at Y (a former work colleague) who is cavorting on the lawn; in fact, he is standing about one meter (3 feet) off the ground and bouncing from tree to tree. He also seems to be walking up in the air … As he wants to show that he is flying for real, he is jumping up really high and keeps flying. I see he has two large white wings. I watch him flying between two trees and find this graceful and beautiful.

In conjunction with all of that, my partner wants to write a letter to someone from Poland. He buys a few items in a store and gives both the letter and his shopping to a big man in a wheelchair.

Dialogue between two parts of the dream.

I decided to initiate a dialogue between Y (the Angel) and the man in a wheelchair (the Cripple), as their capacity to be on the move is totally opposite.

The Angel: *I think you are in a very bad shape and very down-to-earth!*

The man: *For myself, I think you are really crazy! I cannot believe you are actually able to fly and you are a real angel!*

The Angel: *I am not an angel, but I can actually fly! Only fear or believing I can't do it can make me fall down.*

The man: *In any case, I feel firmly rooted to the ground, because I can't even walk. Moving is difficult in itself. In the end, flying would be a lot more convenient for me than for you! Can you teach me?*

The Angel: *Yes, I can, if you really want to learn how. But I think you're far too skeptical to believe you can do it. What do you want with me in this dream?*

The man: *I am the part of you that keeps you grounded! With me, you cannot soar high up in the sky. Let's say I keep you in the real world! I will not allow you to fly so high that you lose touch with reality.*

The Angel: *I am starting to get it. It basically means that the two of us together would neither be flying, nor sitting in a wheel-chair, but just walking. But I do want to keep flying!*

The man: *I am not saying you should stop flying. I would love to fly too! I am telling you not to fly so high that you lose touch with reality!*

The Angel: *But what would I get from not flying as high up?*

The man: *You could at least fly occasionally! Now, do not forget that I am there too and that I can't move fast in a wheelchair!*

I am slowing you down. If you will only accept me as being a part of you, you will be able to fly and I will be able to move forward more easily. In fact, we will both be able to be on the move instead of being stationary! I wish I could walk and stop moving in a wheelchair.

This dream takes up the theme of the ability to be progressing psychologically: On the one hand, the Angel, the part of me that is able to fly, in other words to dream big and develop major projects, and on the other hand, the man in a wheelchair, that is to say, the part of me that moves slowly or with great effort and because of being too down-to-earth, rejects the other aspect of my personality. Harmoniously integrating these two parts of me would help me move forward instead of being paralyzed by the conflict between the two.

Jungian Dialogue with Dream Figures

This method is very similar to the previous one, except for a fundamental aspect: There is no identification with the character of the dream chosen for the dialogue. I recommend it when you (i.e. your conscious self/"I") want to converse with one part of the dream, as opposed to a dialogue between two elements.

Unlike the Gestaltist Perls, Jung (1976) considered that the elements of a dream contain information not only from our personal unconscious; he has shown through his clinical work that archetypal images from the collective unconscious frequently arise. As previously explained, an archetype is some kind of universal pattern found in all cultures throughout the course of history. Therefore, archetypal images belong to the human psyche. These images are somehow rooted in our psychic genetic inheritance. It is found everywhere, but in slightly different forms, because they are influenced by the particular aspects of the culture where they manifest (for more information on archetypes, please refer to Chapter 1).

These images are not exclusively ours; they represent both universal and personal aspects. This is why identifying with a character is inconsistent with this approach, as there is always this danger of an inflated ego by identifying with universal elements which are actually beyond us. In other words, we have to be careful to avoid *peacocking*, as mentioned in Chapter 2. The purpose of the dialogue will be to bring out from the symbols the aspects that are personal to us and can teach something about our life.

The dialogue often takes on the form of questions that bring into focus which part of us is revealed by the symbols, and what this part is telling us in a dream. In a way, it is a fruitful dialogue with the unconscious mind that allows it to speak up freely. The basis of this method is to ask questions, then to listen to the answers that arise from the unconscious mind, without trying to control it, and finally, to let our conscious mind provide answers to the unconscious mind. It is a real dialogue on an equal basis between the unconscious mind and the conscious mind.

Description of the Method

Step #1: Identifying one element of a dream to initiate a dialogue with
Step #2: Writing down the dialogue
Step #3: Identifying the existential message

Step #1: Identifying One Element of a Dream to Initiate a Dialogue With

As a partner in dialogue, please choose someone or something that you basically find intriguing or that you just do not understand. It may even be your own image in the dream. The purpose of the Jungian method is to enable communication with inner figures. Included in that is any part of the dream (even an object) you want to directly initiate a dialogue with rather than through another character, since that would fall under the Gestalt dialogue explained previously.

The Jungian method is more appropriate than the Gestalt dialogue when a dream features archetypal images such as characters who possess great wisdom, a divine or royal aspect or who are highly spiritual in nature. It is also more suited for figures which have a particularly negative aspect, in which case the Gestalt identification approach would cause so much suffering that it would not be of any help whatsoever. For example, if a slimy green horrifying monster arises, you would rather ask questions to find out what he represents and the reason for this form, rather than identifying with it. However, as indicated before, even the Jungian dialogue involves risks. I will come back to this later.

Step #2: Writing Down the Dialogue

This involves asking questions to the character or element of the dream, then listening to the answers that come up and taking note of them. Writing is important as it provides immediate feedback, which allows you to capture the impact of the answers and to stay focused on the dialogue.

The greatest challenge is to avoid fabricating an answer and to make sure you simply listen to the answers that emerge from the core of your being. It requires a bit of practice, as our conscious mind is so used to manage inner experiences that it never keeps quiet! How do you know whether you have made up a satisfactory answer rather than listened to your unconscious mind? If an answer comes as a surprise to you, it is a good indication it is genuine. In general, if the dialogue leads to some kind of insight, such as understanding the meaning of some experience which until then had remained elusive or a strong emotion such as deep joy, deep sadness, anger or frustration, it means you really got in touch with your unconscious mind and you let it speak up. Sometimes, however, the reaction is more subtle: Lessening tension, sighs of relief or a sense of satisfaction following the dialogue. Just see for yourself.

Once you let the unconscious speak through the inner figure, the conscious "I" must respond, react and voice its objections (Johnson, 2009/1986). The conscious "self/I" has a vital role to play. By voicing its objections and disagreements, it keeps us from falling prey to an almighty unconscious mind; the conscious "I" sustains the path of reason, states opposing views, which makes it possible to reach a new balance. The unconscious mind's perspective remains essential and too often ignored; but it is equally important for the conscious mind to play its moderating role of the unconscious mind's impulses. This is the true meaning of a real dialogue between the two, one that creates a new balance of power.

Robert Johnson (1986) warns us against the powerful brute forces of the unconscious mind. He points out that if the dialogue leads to drop all our scruples, our commitments and our responsibilities, and to be in conflict with our family, our friends and our coworkers, then something is out of balance and the conscious "self/I" must regain control. When the "I" and the inner figure are done with fighting and have said all they needed to say, some resolution is occurring. Johnson invites us to continue the dialogue until this resolution takes place, even if repetition is needed. He also stresses the importance to avoid going from one inner figure to another until this resolution has taken place; in other words, we must have discipline, avoid letting our mind wander and continue dialoguing with a single figure of the dream until it is over.

To initiate a dialogue, develop questions from what you find intriguing about the character or object from the dream. The following questions may serve as a guide:

- Who are you?
- Why is it that you look like that?
- What does your life look like?
- Why are you in my dream?
- Do you embody an aspect of me?
- Do you have any message for me?

Just add any other question that sparks a curiosity in you.

Step #3: Identifying the Existential Message

As in the other experiential methods, this step is to briefly point out the existential message of the dream. Usually, it appears quite clearly after such a dialogue. It is helpful to summarise it in a clear and concise sentence.

Application Example

The Angry Dead Man

I am with my life partner and a man dressed in black who is angry.

Step #1: Identifying One Element of a Dream to Initiate a Dialogue With

Intrigued by this angry man dressed in black, I made the decision to converse with him.

Step #2: Writing Down the Dialogue

Dreamer:	*Mr. Man in Black, who are you?*
A man in black:	*I am a tall and lean man, dressed in black, silent, I feel very angry; I am both alive and dead and I remind you of your former spouse.*
Dreamer:	*Are you a part of me?*
A man in black:	*You are well aware that I am!*
Dreamer:	*Which part of me are you?*
A man in black:	*I am the part of you that is tempted to contact your former spouse, a relationship that is dead but still alive.*
Dreamer:	*Why are you angry?*
A man in black:	*Because you are tempted to get closer to me, but you pretend I am not even here. You too are still angry.*
Dreamer:	*Are you telling me I should deal with my anger?*
A man in black:	*Yes, I am.*
Dreamer:	*But why? What could I possibly get out of paying attention to my anger? I think it is really over and it should stay that way.*
A man in black:	*Maybe it could teach you important issues about your current marriage!*
Dreamer:	*Now that is a good reason. I agree to revisit my life experience regarding this past relationship, but I am refusing to contact my former spouse.*

Step #3: Identifying the Existential Message

The message is the following: *I can refuse to see my former spouse again if I want to, but getting in touch with my life experience regarding him could be beneficial for my current marriage.*

Three weeks after this dreamwork, I wrote the following in my dream journal:

Lots of memories of my first marriage are coming back these days. Instead of pushing them away, I realise that I allow them to emerge. Now there were lots of issues to address about my first marriage. I find it valuable that my dream and the ensuing dialogue enabled me to distinguish between "getting in touch with my former spouse" and "getting in touch with my life experience" regarding this marriage, which can be important for my current marital union.

Two months later, my former spouse I had not seen for seven years contacted me to hear from me! I made the decision to meet him. We were able to talk about what had happened between us and to say what was left unsaid back then.

Exploring the Sounds and Movements of a Dream

The following is a method, original in every respect, developed by Mrs. Michelle Rinfret, a French-Canadian psychologist. Mrs. Rinfret considers approaching the psyche through the body as a powerful means. This method evolved quite naturally from her interest, since movements and sounds are effective ways of bodily expression. The only method resembling the one developed by Mrs. Rinfret is the Jungian Dance-Movement Therapy from Mrs. Mary Whitehouse. This approach uses images and dreaming experience as catalysts for spontaneous movement; the specific content of the dream is thus expressed through movement (See Zwig, 1991). Mrs. Rinfret's method is in some way different, though, as it uses sounds as well. Here is what she says about it:

> *This approach has an active dimension. At any time, the body is directly involved in the action, which makes the experience very real. One is less likely to get lost into wild imagining about the experience. This direct and immediate access to oneself encourages involvement in the experience for the individual who is examining himself through dreaming (Rinfret, 1992).*

About sounds, she specifies that reluctance to express them seems even greater than for movements. This channel of self-expression seems to have been even more overlooked in occidental culture. It has become more secret, more hidden and less known, even for oneself. One must familiarise with it and let it awaken gradually. During familiarising exercises, one participant was yawning repeatedly and tears were running down her cheeks while she was feeling no particular emotion. Later on, a couple of memories from her youth came back. "It seems like it impacts another memory, she says. It is both frightening and appealing." *(Rinfret, 1992).*

This approach can be used by oneself at home, but also in a group; in this instance, the group's participants play different roles from a dream, much like the well-known method *Theater of dreams*. About her method used in groups, Mrs. Rinfret says the following:

> *It is wonderful to notice that the group participants play each in turn a house, a male or female co-worker, a landscape or even a chair. In fact, the latter case illustrates clearly the vibrant dimension taken on by the acted images. In one group, warm support was received by a participant who was lying on an imaginary chair whose armrests, headrest and footrest were actually living people! (Rinfret, 1992).*

You may feel reluctant to use movements and sounds to explore dreams. However, having reluctances can help identify how your self-expression is restricted. The following description will help you see how this method can be applied.

Description of the Method

Step #1: Identifying kinesthetic and sound elements
Step #2: Generating movements and sounds physically
Step #3: Completing movements and sounds
Step #4: Identifying the existential message

Step #1: Identifying Kinesthetic and Sound Elements

This step is simply a matter of identifying the movements and sounds either made by yourself or other characters from a dream; these can be people, animals or objects.

Step #2: Generating Movements and Sounds Physically

Starting with the most obvious, the most intriguing or the most fascinating one, emulate the movements in the dream with your body, within space. If you make sounds as well, just make them along with the movements. As you go along, it is important to observe your responses to the movements and sounds you make. Do you find it pleasant, unpleasant, frustrating, strange, new, scary? Mentally note all your reactions without censoring them. If possible, and if you feel comfortable with this, use a mirror while doing it.

Step #3: Completing Movements and Sounds

Once you have emulated the movements in the dream, ask yourself which ones are incomplete, partial or interrupted and repeat them so as to complete them all. You can also consider which movements would be more satisfactory if they were done differently; physically emulate any altered movement. Therefore, it is a matter of experimenting new movements just to see how your body is impacted and consequently your life experience. Most of dreams remain unfinished or end in an unsatisfactory manner; that is why completing them generally provides useful clues for identifying the existential message associated with a dream. The same questions should be asked concerning sounds: Are the sounds too low or incomplete? Does it feel uncomfortable to generate sounds? If so, pay attention to what you experience when you are generating sounds, and respect any reluctance to do so, because this method is a very powerful one!

Mrs. Rinfret warns us against a number of pitfalls:

- Do not invest in miming or in theatrics to the expense of your inner feelings;
- Avoid reducing the impact of sound and movement by getting lost in a lot of explanations;
- Be mindful not to downplay the importance of the dreamer by too much involvement from the other participants in a group.

Step #4: Identifying the Existential Message

As for the other methods, please take a few moments to make a short sentence stating the existential message from the dream, as currently understood. In the first place, you may feel the need to take note of your reactions during the experience so that the existential message can emerge from it. The following questions can help you state the message:

- Which movements do I feel like completing further? What is it revealing about what needs to be completed in my life?
- Which movements are new to me, and are they bringing something new to my life?
- Are there sounds that are repressed? Is there anything incomplete in my self-expression? Is there anything left unsaid that I now feel like saying?
- Does the dream teach me anything new about how I feel in my life?

Please add any other question that is challenging for you and helps you identify the existential message from the dream.

Application Example

A 40-year-old woman had the following dream:

An Encounter with a Cow

I am looking at a cow that is holding still under an outdoor shelter. It is neither very tall nor very fat. It is spotted black and white. I am staring at the cow's udder in particular, thinking that I would like to milk it. Dare I try while there is nobody around to teach me how? I see myself squeezing my fingers on the cow's teats. I once heard that it takes strength to milk a cow. Will I be strong enough? I must also be careful not to hurt the cow, because this is a very sensitive part of the body when it is full of milk. I seems to me that I can be both efficient and careful. As I skip around, I leave and say to the cow: "I will be back tomorrow when you are full of milk."

Step #1: Identifying Kinesthetic and Sound Elements

The sounds and movements are the following:

- *The cow is holding still (no movement);*
- *The eyes are moving to stare at the udder;*
- *There is an imaginary movement, to milk the cow;*
- *I am skipping around;*
- *I am talking to the cow.*

Step #2: Generating Movements and Sounds Physically

For me, the second step takes place along with the third one.

Step #3: Completing Movements and Sounds

Holding still, I imagine that I am staring at the cow that is also motionless. I feel inner stillness due to this encounter of two motionless beings. The black and white spots and the big eyes of the cow hold my attention. Leaving questions behind, I take action.

Using both my hands, I recreate the grasping movement to squeeze the teats of the imaginary cow with strength and carefulness in order to extract milk. I may be a city farmer, but I am doing pretty well! I am gradually getting into my own pace and building a cadence. I am humming. I feel happy. I have fun imitating the hissing sound of milk flowing into the bucket. Images keep coming to mind and I re-experience the bliss I felt when I was breastfeeding. I imagine that I am gratefully drinking the warm milk from the bucket.

To drink, to take. To eat. I fancy becoming the cow. I get down on all fours. My breasts are sagging. Erotic fantasies. To have sex. To give. Staying immersed into the dream, I alternately get on all fours and sit to milk the cow and drink. I start dancing with delight. I get up and keep on dancing, feeling grateful.

Step #4: Identifying the Existential Message

This work puts me in touch with the sharing circle. I am given permission to take more, to eat more food and to nurture my erotic life specifically.

Dream Re-entry

The re-entry method is inspired from Carl Jung; he sometimes asked his clients to use *active imagination* to further the dream story. This approach enables to explore one's inner images and to initiate a dialogue with different unconscious parts of oneself (Johnson, 2009/1986). Involvement is required from the ego that initiates an active and conscious dialogue through emotions and feelings, which is contrary to passive fantasies. The ego talks, discusses and interacts with inner imaginary images. These images, "They talk about things you never consciously knew and express thoughts that you never consciously thought". (Johnson, 1986, p. 138) This experience is real, involves actual feelings and has the power to change anybody who is engaged in it. It can help harmonise conflicted parts of oneself and create inner peace. As active imagination is a very powerful approach, it might be appropriate to seek help from a trusted professional experienced in this method. If you use active imagination by your-self and feel helpless, please stop before going any further.

Re-entry into a dream is often suggested in connection with nightmares by several authors. However, this approach may apply to any dream whose par-ticular atmosphere or mysterious images you wish to further explore in order to better grasp the existential message. For example, if images from a dream require continuing exploration, such as a cave with something of interest or a treasure chest, it is appropriate to enter into the cave on an imaginary journey or to open the treasure chest in order to discover its contents. In doing so, you are entering into the underground realm of dreaming, a phrase from Hillman (1979) who suggests leaving rational thought behind in order to explore further dream images and see where they lead.

For dream re-entry, return to the dream's background in order to review how it unfolds and go back to the last image of the dream. Just pay close attention to what is spontaneously unfolding in your imagination beyond where it ended, such as what the characters say or do, how the dream scenes shift and how you respond and interact with the dream figures. You might want to wait before writing about what happened. It is important to actively interact by asking questions to the dream figures, to express what you think and to possibly make counter arguments to what is suggested while letting your imagination leading the scenes. Do not try to control what is coming, just be actively involved by genuinely sharing your response to what happens.

Similarly, some authors (see *Collectif de l'arc-en-ciel*, 1991) suggests surren-dering to what happens. For example, allow yourself to fall backwards if you are about to, to be caught by whoever is chasing you, and observe any devel-opment. It is important to let your imagination spontaneously do its thing. You can start by asking one question or by responding to a figure from the dream.

Application Example

A 56-year-old woman had the following dream:

Three Women with Blue Dresses

I see three prostitutes in a house with a number of bedrooms. Two women are 20 years old and the third one is 30 years old. Each one is wearing a shimmering blue dress with jewelry sewn into. They are also wearing necklaces and look like long-necked African women, only their neck has a normal length and a normal size. They look gorgeous in their dresses. The 30-year-old woman is dignified, sweet and more collected.

Intrigued by these women, the dreamer made the decision to use the re-entry approach into the dream. She started with asking the three women what they meant to tell her in this dream. Then she saw the following images and a dialogue took place in her imagination as follows:

The *three women took her by the hand and started dancing in circles. While they were dancing, they got her the same blue dress and the same jewelry, telling her she was the fourth woman. Then the male clients came in and the women had to take care of them. They wanted to leave her with a client, but the dreamer felt outraged and refused. Then the oldest woman, the third one, explained that they were priestesses to Aphrodite, the Goddess of Love and Pleasure, not prostitutes.*

The dreamer realised that the existential message was to connect better to her own sensuality and to tell her partner clearly what she enjoys in sexual relations.

5
Art Therapy
Dreamwork Methods

I consider art as a preferred method to elucidate a dream's message, mainly because it enables an image's evocative power to work its magic.

Very often, the mere fact of reproducing a dream's image causes completely unexpected and eye-opening effects. The existential message might become immediately apparent, simply because the image can be contemplated in great detail. You might also feel a deep sense of peace just because you actually breathed life into an inner reality. Recreating the image in three dimensions has even more striking impacts. Carl Jung (1993) wrote that giving shape to an image from the unconscious mind is therapeutic in itself. This was confirmed by my own experience. Madeline McMurray's book (1988) masterfully illustrates the healing power of images.

Art actually allows expressing the evolution of our life experience at any moment, because our artistic expression reflects our dynamic inner reality through our hands.

This chapter describes four art therapy methods for dreamwork, by means of drawing or painting, a three-dimensional reproduction, drawing a dream's elusive sensation and quick sketches to help easing nightmares. Each method works with the same three steps, which might apply with slight differences depending on its specificity. These steps will first be explained in general terms, followed with detailed explanations on each of the four individual art therapy dreamwork methods.

Three Common Steps for the Art Therapy Dreamwork Methods

Step #1: Exploring dream images through an art medium
Step #2: Finding meaning in the art experience through writing
Step #3: Identifying the existential message

Step #1: Exploring Dream Images Through an Art Medium

There is no need to know how to paint, draw or have experience with art media to benefit from the full impact of this step. The mere act of visually translating into colors, lines and shapes the *primordial image* or impression of a dream as a whole promotes the awareness of aspects that otherwise would have remained unnoticed. This work also brings out the emotional reaction, the very one we need to understand the meaning of a dream.

A dream's *primordial image* is the one that sticks in your mind when you think back to a dream; it usually is the most striking for you. Indeed, you will observe that when remembering a dream, an image, a sound or a particular feeling systematically arises, rather than evocative words, except for those few occasions where only a few strong words are left. This is what is meant by a dream's *primordial image*, the word "image" having a broad sense.

The importance of the evocative power of images was explained previously. Giving images a physical reality by means of drawing, painting or other media allows to reveal their full impact. These explorations through art provide access to a deep experience you may subsequently write about at Step #2, and this process will help you go further.

Step #2: Finding Meaning in the Art Experience Through Writing

Now that a drawing or a painting was created, it is useful to put words on it to easily elucidate the meaning of your dream. In the next pages, I suggest three written exercises to put into words the lived experience at Step #1 about exploring the dream through art. With these exercises, you will recognise, among other things, the methods of identification and dialogue already explained in the previous chapter, but now adapted to complement the plastic artwork productions suggested in the art therapy methods.

Reactions and Spontaneous Associations to Artwork

Very often, our reactions to artwork production and all that we went through while creating offer all the information needed to elucidate a dream's existential message. The mere act of reproducing a dream's image with art materials causes a wide range of reactions. It also causes spontaneous associations with the image that appears before our eyes. All these reactions are not pulled out of thin air; they are loaded with unexpected clues about the meaning of the dream. That is why, at this stage, any spontaneous reaction should be noted so that you can draw the appropriate conclusions thereafter. What is worth noting in particular? Anything that prompted a response during artwork creation may have meaning; the following is a non-exhaustive list.

You may take note of your reactions to:

- A part of the drawing or the plastic artwork production you dislike;
- On the contrary, a part you particularly like;
- Different types of lines and shapes;
- The colors you used and how they impact you;
- The images that appear, even if they are different from what the dream inspired;
- The overall impression that is conveyed; for example, a figure that is strayed in a large white space gives rise to some fears in you, or on the contrary brings a sense of comfort, or a creepy mask feels frightening, etc.;
- The medium that was used (gouache, dry pastels, oil pastels, felt-tip pens, finger paint, watercolors, modeling clay, fabrics, or other materials) and any sensation caused by these mediums, such as satisfaction, frustration, etc.;
- Any other reaction you might have had during the creative process.
- The dream's existential message may well arise from these brief notes.

Identification to Images

You can also identify with a drawn or painted image from a dream, which is a Gestalt technique. The following written tool, as well as the next one, were developed in collaboration with my colleague, Lorraine Dumont, a psychologist and art therapist. After producing an image from the dream, use writing to identify yourself with the image, as follows:

- Describe the image as well as the impression that emerges from it, as precisely as possible, using qualifiers, as if you were trying to explain it to someone who does not see it. It is not a matter of rewriting the whole dream, but of distancing yourself from it to describe only the image or object that is now in front of you.
- Read your writings again, assuming for a moment that it accurately describes a current aspect of yourself or your life. Take note of any reaction to this experience.
- Complete the following sentences, choosing from among these:
  - Thanks to you, I am becoming aware that I am …
  - I now feel …
  - I am deciding that …

Dialoguing with Images

The Jungian dialogue is another way of working on an image from a dream after having reproduced it through artwork. This is a particularly appropriate method when the meaning of a dream remains elusive, or when a dream carries archetypal figures, in other words very impressive figures either positive or negative, since it makes it possible to avoid identifying with it directly, which may often cause discomfort.

It is about asking questions, then listening to the answers that come up and then writing them down. The greatest challenge is to avoid fabricating an answer, and to make sure to listen to the answers emerging from the core of your being. As mentioned earlier, if an answer comes as a surprise to you, it is a sign that you are on the right track.

The following questions may serve as a guide:

- Who are you?
- Why is it that you look like that?
- What does your life look like?
- Why are you in my dream?
- Do you embody an aspect of me?
- Do you have any message for me?
- Any other question you are curious about.

Step #3: Decoding the Existential Message

Once you have reproduced or created a dream's image and noted what you experienced, all you have to do is to word the dream's existential message in a short sentence. Although it often contains wisdom applicable to human life as a whole, an existential message is useful to the extent that it relates to a specific situation in your current life. At this point, your graphic creation and writings should have allowed to make a connection between the events or concerns in your waking life and the symbols from the dream.

Four Art Therapy Dreamwork Methods

Drawing or Painting a Dream

Once you have chosen the image to represent, it is simply a matter of leaving it up to your hand to spontaneously create, using lines, shapes and colors. Color in particular is a key element, as the color choice which best reflects the atmosphere related to the dream's image can be decisive to raise awareness of the message. What if you do not recall seeing any colors in your dream? It is not that important. Just draw asking yourself what shade or color scheme seems to best reflect the impression from the image. If you are hesitating between a number of different colors, just try several ones to find out which one is appropriate.

Use lines in the same way: What kind of line accurately reflects that particular image and at what pace? A simple line contains a whole world in itself, since the gesture used to trace it may be enough to raise awareness about events remaining unconscious. For example, tracing a line with anger does not require the same gesture nor the same energy as a line traced with gentleness; it is therefore likely to bring back repressed or denied anger, which might be conveyed in a particular dream.

What shape accurately reflects the image? Is it a circle, a square, a rectangle? Just stick with simple shapes, since an approximation is good enough to understand what it is about.

Art Materials

For a two-dimensional work, like a drawing or a painting, let's have in hand paper sheets, pencils and paint. The size of the paper sheets makes a difference, as it is important to have plenty of space. Paper sheets of 46 cm × 61 cm/ 18" × 24" are suitable for self-expression; with smaller paper sheets though, you may feel restricted. The important thing is to trust your instincts and respect your preferences. Different dreams may require the use of paper sheets of a different size. It is up to you. For example, carving the sea monster from your worst nightmare can be a traumatic experience on a large paper sheet, but stimulate discovery in a smaller format, since the monster's terrifying appearance will seem less threatening.

The art medium selected for artwork is equally important. Ideally, a large selection of art media is recommended. First get oil pastels as they are both inexpensive and easy to use. If you do not like their texture, try chalk pastels; a box of twelve sticks of different colors will do, but it is always better to have as wide a variety of colors as possible. You will find boxes of 48 different colors of both pastel types.

Here is the selection I suggest:

- Wooden pencils, wax crayons or felt-tip pens. They are very well suited for drawings about anxiety dreams or for getting control over one's emotions because they are easy to use: Clear and precise lines are easily traced and colors are non-smudging.
- Oil pastels. They too allow for better control but also for more nuances, because of the particular greasy texture of the pencils.
- Chalk/dry pastels. Favorites for some, they are a mix of the above dry mediums and liquid mediums like paint. Their powdery texture is particularly suitable for soft and ethereal moods, mysterious atmospheres as well as blurred shapes. They are not recommended for reproducing specific shapes when details of the drawing matter.
- Gouache (tempera). It is opaque and thick, with very bright colors. Colors can be mixed to produce new shades. This art medium helps to highlight the essence of the feelings present in a dream. While it is difficult to control because the paint does not always produce the desired effect, may smudge

or produce unexpected results, it can bring out some unconscious aspect with more clarity. Gouache and liquid mediums are usually not recommended for drawings on terrifying dreams or anxiety dreams because these require mediums easier to control.

- Watercolor or water-based paint. In cakes or tubes, this type of paint is even more difficult to control. You have to be prepared to make the most of the fluid qualities of watercolor to appreciate this medium. Watercolor beautifully renders the ambiance featured in a dream as well as any blurred impressions and vague sensations; it helps to clarify the realm of feelings of a dream.
- Finger paint. The most difficult medium to control, finger paint instantaneously gives rise to any strong emotions and sensations in the dream. It is ideal to reflect primitive or regressive dimensions, downright sensual aspects or raw emotions. The use of finger paint comes down to dipping one's fingers into the unconscious mind to bring into focus a dimension that is often quite unexpected!

Application Example

Step #1: Exploring the primordial image of a dream through an art medium

The Eggs (see Figure 3)

I see myself ripping apart a rockfall made of huge rocks. Below, I find a big dead crow, all black, lying next to a nest with four big eggs. Two eggs are open and their egg yolks have spilled over. One of other egg is cracked and the fourth one is whole. These two look like the smaller eggs from another nest I saw before, only bigger.

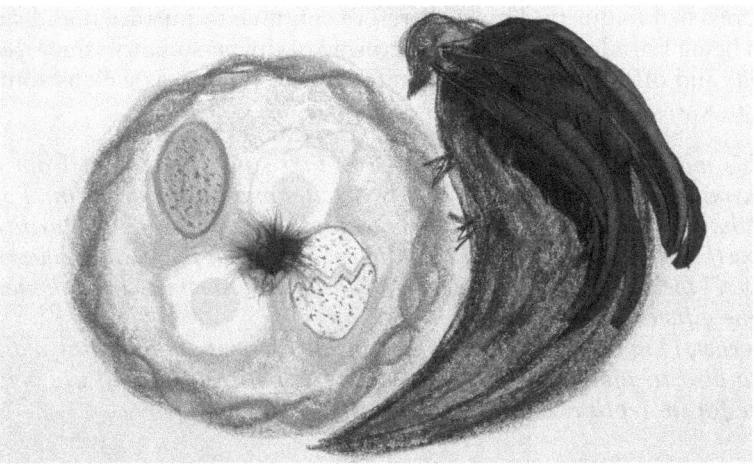

Figure 5.1 *The Eggs.* 46 × 61 cm/18" × 24", chalk pastels and feathers. Photograph Credit: Michelle Boulay, Sherbrooke, Qc. Canada.

Step #2: Finding meaning in the art experience through writing

When I was drawing the nest, I noted the following reactions and associations:

- *The two broken eggs basically become two eggs over-easy ready to be eaten. Therefore, I have food to eat.*
- *After completing the drawing, I added two black feathers to the bird and one small brown feather in the middle of the nest. The addition of black feathers immediately brings to mind a grieving process.*
- *The four eggs, open or whole, remind me at once of a mandala[1], especially since the circular shape is featured on the outer edge of the nest. This impression is confirmed when I spontaneously add a small feather at the center of the nest.*
- *In addition, this small feather reminds me of a newborn small bird. Once drawn, the cracked egg brings to mind an Easter egg; it is not open and dried as I first thought, but whole, closed and even decorated. It reminds me of gifts, joy and celebrations.*
- *On the left side, the whole egg has not quite reached maturity; I can tell by its size. However reluctantly, I have drawn it in a smaller size and I immediately felt bothered. I felt disturbed by that because the dead crow will not sit on her egg so that it grows to maturity. I take comfort in knowing that it is something I can "sit on" for myself and take care of in order to help it reach maturity.*

Step #3: Decoding the existential message

Here is a summary of what I understand from this: Something in me has died; I am mourning something even though I do not know yet what it is about. The mourning comes along with something new that has just been born but has not reached maturity; I must therefore continue to nurture it and sit on it. What is being born looks like a restructuring of my personality (since there is a mandala) and offers nurturing, joy and surprises for me, as well as something else yet unknown.

Does this make sense to me or not? Does that sound like what I am feeling in my waking life these days? Actually, I felt something new in me lately; at times, I have the feeling of being able to find my own presence nurturing, to love myself better, whereas before I did not know what it meant to love oneself. Moreover, I feel that all this is still fragile and that it must be strengthened. This brings me gifts of joy and surprises!

However, I am wondering what died inside of me. I am initiating a dialogue with the bird to understand what it is about. This time, I will use a Jungian dialogue for in-depth exploration of my dream.

---

[1]   As mentioned earlier, "mandala" means magic circle in Sanscrit; it usually is a circle with a centre divided into four, eight, twelve or even sixteen sections. See Jung, 1972.

Return to Step #2: Finding meaning in the art experience through writing: A Jungian dialogue

– *Who are you, dead bird?*
– *I am a mama-bird who died under a rockfall of very heavy rocks before I was finished with incubating my eggs.*
– *It reminds me of a part of myself that may not have had time to fully develop, because of being buried under something too heavy. Is that what you represent?*
– *Yes, absolutely.*
– *Do you also represent something that is dying in me right now?*
– *Yes, the heaviness and the pain associated with what had not been completed.*

Return to Step #3: Decoding the existential message

In summary, for me the existential message of this dream is the following: A heavy and painful part of me is now dying, and love for myself is being born, although it is still fragile and needs being taken care of.

All of this makes so much sense to me! And how reassuring it is, because it clearly identifies something I have been feeling in a more or less confused way that has now become clear.

Three-Dimensional Reproduction of a Dream Object

To my knowledge, only Patricia Garfield (1999) and Jill Mellick (2001, 1996) suggested the possibility of three-dimensional reproduction of dreams. This idea, however, is not new. The Senoi people, whom I did briefly speak about, reproduced the paintings, the music or the art objects that emerged in dreams. The variation of this method that is suggested here was first taught to me by Lillian Rhinehart and Paula Engelhorn, two art-therapists from California. Mrs. Lorraine Dumont, art therapist from Montréal, and myself added the written exercises.

This method may be used right after a drawing or a painting related to a dream, or be used independently. The three-dimensional reproduction of a dream helps the individual understand its message more deeply and to get in touch with his personal resources and creativity. He can thus go one step further toward solving the existential problem arising from the dream.

For this method, you will need a full selection of art materials. You can start to gather them now. Choose preferably natural objects. The following is a non-exhaustive list:

• Modeling clay;
• Tree branches;

- Pieces of wood planks;
- Leather;
- Rattan;
- Raffia;
- Feathers;
- Shells;
- Pine cones;
- Wool (All rainbow colors: Red, yellow, orange, green, blue, purple, as well as black wool and white wool);
- Fabrics (All rainbow colors: Red, yellow, orange, green, blue, purple, as well as black fabric and white fabric);
- Lace;
- Dried flowers;
- Pebbles;
- Paper sheets of different types: Silk paper, construction paper, glazed paper, wrapping paper, etc.;
- Magazines for paper cutting and collages;
- Threading beads;
- Buttons.

Materials for assembling and cutting will also be needed, like scissors, nails, hammer, glue, sewing thread, needles, among other things.

If you are using this method following any drawing or painting related to a dream, that image will probably become a starting point to reproduce the three-dimensional dream, but not necessarily.

Step #1: Three-Dimensional Reproduction of a Dream's Fragment

Please clearly state in your mind your intention to make a three-dimensional reproduction of your dream, as if you were introducing a program into your inner computer, that is your brain. Then just forget about the program, and let your fingers and your eyes select the textures and colors you find attractive among the available material, without having any particular plan in mind. Once you have collected all the materials, work with them and arrange them so as to build something, letting your hands come and go. At some point, you may get a clear idea of what you want to build, or you may on the contrary not grasp the end result before completion. If a specific piece of art appeared in your dream, you may decide from the start to replicate it.

Step #2: Finding Meaning in the Art Experience Through Writing

To put the lived experience into words, you may use one of the three written exercises suggested in Step #2 of the art therapy dreamwork methods (see the first pages of this chapter). Taking note of any spontaneous reactions while using the materials will probably be the most useful method in the present case, since the mere act of assembling materials will cause a number of significant reactions. Indeed, anything that stirred reactions during art creation might be meaningful. As a reminder, you can take note of your reactions to the following.

- The different types of lines and shapes of the object you are making.
- The colors used and their impact on you.
- The overall impression from your artwork; for example, you may feel dissatisfied with the object or on the contrary get a sense of comfort from it, or if you felt frightened by a mask you created, etc.
- The sensations that arose while you worked: Satisfaction, frustration, etc.
- Any other reaction that might have been stirred during the creative process.

The existential message may indeed emerge by itself from these few notes.

Step #3: Decoding the Existential Message

After the three-dimensional reproduction of a dream's fragment and writing about that experience, the existential message that emerged through writing must be worded in a short sentence. The very creation of the object will probably have brought forth the dream's existential message; the writing stage may not have been even necessary. The mere act of wording the message in clear and specific terms helps to raise awareness about it.

Application Example

The following is a dream that was worked on one month later, just before the woman's 40th birthday.

My White Childlike Circle

I feel the need, like an impulse, to touch something that feels like a White Childlike Circle. It seems that a man does not want me to enter the Circle, but I decide to enter and touch it. I wake up to find my hand on my pubic area, feeling contractions.

Step #1: Three-dimensional reproduction of a dream's fragment

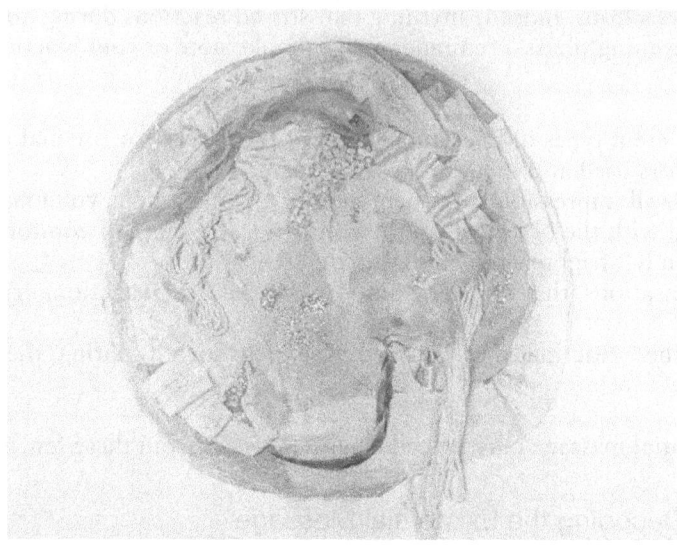

Figure 5.2 *My White Childlike Circle*. Paper, lace, fabric, wool, veil, cotton, silk, Styrofoam ball and feathers.

Step #2: Finding meaning in the art experience through writing

Creating the *White Childlike Circle* that woman saw in her dream led to many different reactions and associations she took note of:

At first, it felt important to reproduce a white circle so as to make it both rich and tangible. I sought to explore the white color in all its nuances and in a variety of textures using paper, lace, fabric, wool, etc. Some contrasts quickly became obvious: There was one between the light, fragile and soft veil and the rougher and warmer wool, and there was another one between the very soft silk and the more textured cotton.

Then I felt something was missing; I picked up a Styrofoam ball, cut it in two and glued it onto the circle. I added white bird feathers, which almost felt like down, and covered the ball with them. That appeared to me to be a small mountain, a mons pubis.

I wrapped around the small mountain a tuft of wool extending out of the frame. This aspect was very important to me, as it represented a less structured and slightly anarchic aspect, something "out of the box". Finally, I added a longer feather as well as confetti and sparkles; it turned into a celebration, a blast, a lot of fun, and it enhanced the whole circle. Then I felt that the process was coming to a close.

My dream referred to an impulse, which I identified while I was working: I was totally immersed in my work and had a lot of energy; this was not only changing, it was also changing me; it felt magical and brought me back to the time when I was making sculptures and weaving. For me, fabrics are palpable, tangible, warm and sensuous.

This experience felt intense, exciting and playful. My own expression both felt liberating, like a culminating point. I was wondering whether this was actually brought out of me, and a sense of awe came over me.

Step #3: Decoding the existential message

Dreamer's comments

I worked on this dream the day before my fortieth birthday. I wanted this celebration to be unique and truly special. On the eve of my birthday, I was able to reach my loved ones by creating exactly the same energy I had felt while creating my White Childlike Circle. As a result, my birthday party was filled with energy, creativity, friendship and love, everything I was open to receive.

That evening, I suggested a game without worrying about what other people would think. So, I allowed spontaneous self-expression, which had always been difficult for me before. I discovered the joy of doing things for free, of being immersed into what I was doing, both during the celebration and for the creation of the circle. I rediscovered the childlike purity and spontaneity, just like the white color that I relate to purity and the circle I relate to a balloon. My creative inner child was in the here and now.

Furthermore, the various textures refer to different sides of me: I am warm, gentle, rough, fragile and real. All I have inside of me and all the different sides of me come together in a harmonious unity and will now express themselves outwardly, as the tuft of wool extending out of the frame; they will spontaneously be expressed.

The existential message could be summarised as follows: I am now a harmonious unity; I want this uniqueness to express itself through my creativity and when I do that, I allow my energy to radiate outward.

I still have unanswered questions because I am not sure how I can successfully take my inner potential forth out into daily life. Moreover, I am currently questioning my career orientation.

Drawing or Painting an Elusive Sensation from a Dream

This method is particularly useful for in-depth exploration of dreams that leave a very strong sensation yet indefinite. In some cases, meditating on the elusive sensation is enough to reveal the dream's message, but it may remain more or less obscure. In this case, lines, shapes and colors are particularly appropriate tools to better explore this vague feeling. Better than words, they may indeed express the vague and abstract sensation from a dream more accurately.

By making visible what you sense using lines, shapes and colors, you have more control over your inner experience. Because the elusive sensation is, by definition, fleeting, this technique works all the better when used upon waking up.

Step #1: Exploring the Elusive Sensation Through Drawing and Painting

In practical terms, it is about using lines, shapes and colors to make an abstract drawing of the feeling that remains unclear. While you are drawing, it is important to stay in touch with the elusive sensation, even if it means to pause from time to time in order to bring it up whenever it slips out of your mind and/or to make sure the drawing or the painting accurately reflects your inner experience or at least comes as close as possible to it. Which lines, shapes and colors best reflect the particular sensation from the dream? You know that you got in touch with it when it comes back strongly just as you use a specific color or trace a specific line or an evocative shape. Your drawing is complete when you run out of inspiration or it feels complete to you.

Step #2: Finding Meaning in the Art Experience Through Writing

Once your drawing or painting is complete, writing about your experience will help find the existential message. You may first describe your drawing or painting as faithfully as possible based on its lines, its colors, its shapes, its movement or else the impression emerging from it. Then you just check whether this description also applies to the elusive sensation that revealed itself.

Step #3: Identifying the Existential Message

Once the elusive sensation becomes clear enough, just ask yourself to which aspect it refers to in your life: Where and when did you feel something similar in your waking life? The answer to this question will lead to the dream's existential message.

If the sensation nevertheless remains somewhat elusive, please just respect the fact that it is a little bit clearer for you: The time has not come yet for the existential message to come to light. The dreamwork accomplished through drawing or painting will not be lost. The same sensation will find its way into another dream, in a somewhat clearer form, and will shift time and time again until it is ready to be totally revealed by the unconscious mind.

Application Example

The Swan's Music

In my dream, I am wondering "How come I do not listen to the swan's music?" *I am immediately left with a very strong feeling of what it would be – an impression of great beauty – and this obviously is what I need to do. For a brief moment, I feel concerned about the expression "The swan's song" which seems to refer to the end of something.*

Dreamer's comments

I first started to meditate on the elusive sensation. I slowly repeated the same question again and again "How come I don't listen to the swan's music?" Then the following images and emotions arose from within me.

- *I am sure that is what I need to do*
- *I feel sereine*
- *The caramel color*
- *I have a feeling that I am finally coming back home*
- *I feel like I am recognising something that sounds familiar to me*
- *I get this instruction: "Listen to the voice of beauty and serenity"*
- *"Listen to that voice from deep within instead of not having confidence in yourself and of listening to the voice of doubt."*

Step #1: Drawing the elusive sensation

I drew this feeling of great beauty using the caramel color that came to mind. I have fun applying this color and similar ones on many paper sheets, using chalk pastels.

Step #2: Identifying the elusive sensation through writing

While I was drawing, it became obvious that a lot of gentleness was suggested through my creation, both through the swan's shape and the color I used.

Step #3: Identifying the existential message

What I understood from the existential message is that I have to treat myself with much gentleness and to love myself more! I also took good note of the idea of listening from deep within instead of always doubting myself. Isn't it another way of loving myself?

Practical Applications

As a hands-on activity, I decided to look for music works on the swan's song. I also intended to meditate on what might be coming to an end in my life, because of the brief concern felt at the end of the dream. What was likely drawing to a close was the feeling of being an ugly duckling! This made sense given that at the time when I had this dream, I had been in a rewarding relationship for the last seven years. It appears that in a couple, it takes seven years for a partner who feels insecure in relationships to move to a trustful attachment form, in other words to a more peaceful relationship (Hass-Cohen and Clyde-Findlay, 2015).

Now, shortly after completing the dreamwork, I listened to The Swan by Saint-Saëns and Swan Lake by Tchaikovsky. The latter seemed familiar and I was pleased to hear it again, since I had been ice skating with that music in my teen years. As for Tchaikovsky's music, it was of particular interest to me: It seemed filled with tenderness and it once again confirmed the existential message I was getting.

Finally, I went back to "The eggs" dream (previously in this chapter) and I got clues about what was dying: A heavy and painful side of me which was already much lighter and healthy at the time I had the Swan's music dream.

This image of the swan had been with me for some time. Seven years before (see Chapter 1), I had the dream "The swan with burned off wings"; that image helped me discover I was not satisfied with my decision of the time, because the swan had burned off wings. This time, the swan was doing much better and was inviting me to trust him even more. Even today, I pay close attention to this personal dreaming symbol when it comes up in my dreams.

Quick Sketch to Appease a Nightmare

As was already explained in Chapter 1, a nightmare is a symbolic dream which can leave highly intense feelings of fear, terror or anxiety upon waking up. Typically, the dreamer is being chased hostilely by a human, an animal figure or a monster, or he feels helpless because of life threatening situations like suffocation, falling down through the air, drowning, paralysis, loss of control, feeling lost or humiliated in public (for example, failing an exam in public.) Nightmares can also be about traumas with images depicting past traumatic experiences, like a car accident, a war scene (for veterans) or any other event about threats of death or injury. Nightmares are very important for our personal growth as they offer an opportunity for working on many traumatic or unconscious aspects.

The first thing to do upon waking up from a nightmare is to work on easing the painful emotion. To do so, you may first look for the area where it is felt in your body. Is it in your heart? In your chest? In your belly? Is there a sense of fear, horror, terror, panic, imminent threat, an intense feeling of loss, mourning, the world coming to an end, hopelessness, suffering, powerfulness, vulnerability, betrayal, guilt? Does it go along with painful sensations like shortness of breath, sweating, rapid heartbeats or pains?

Then start breathing, that is to say inhaling then exhaling as described below, and you will calm down very quickly. As you inhale, just think the following: "I presently have feelings of fear (or horror, terror, panic or any other emotion that comes to mind)"; then as you exhale, repeat the following mantra in your mind: "I am letting go of fear (horror, terror, panic or any other emotion that comes to mind)". Repeat as many times as necessary, but it usually does not take too long. This technique is inspired by the mindfulness meditation (Kabat-Zinn, 2009). In the following chapter about lucid dreaming, this type of meditation is described in more detail (Gagliardi, 2016).

Afterwards, you can make a quick and rough color drawing of the emotion using a dry medium. You may also choose to represent the painful physical sensation on a quickly drafted human figure. This step is extremely effective

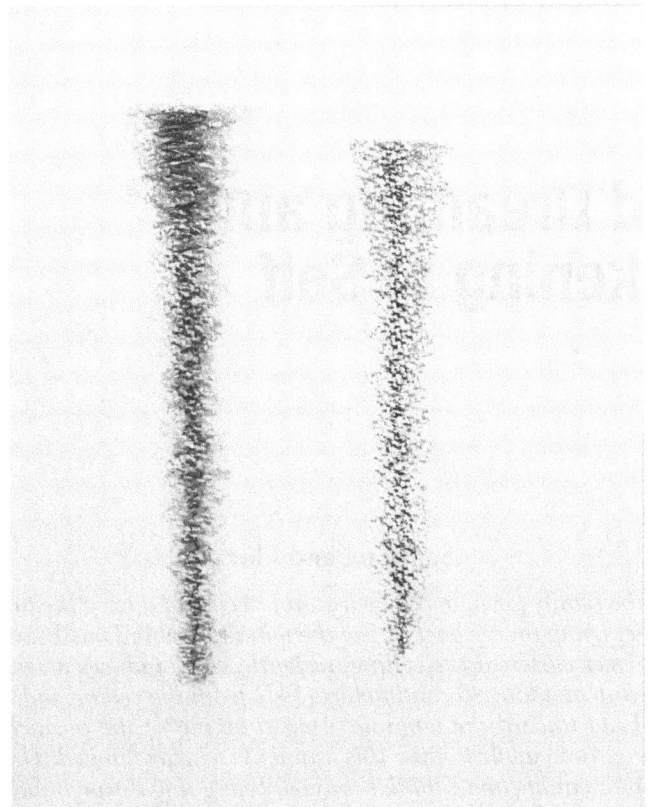

Figure 5.3 *Quick Sketch About Sadness.* 21½ × 27½ cm/8½" × 11". Oil pastels.
Photograph Credit: Michelle Boulay, Sherbrooke, Qc. Canada.

to ease painful emotions and sensations. For example, upon waking up from a nightmare, I was feeling very sad. After a quick sketch about this feeling (see Figure 5.3), I immediately calmed down. I was able to get back to sleep after noting down the nightmare, knowing I could come back to it a few days later to understand what the sadness feeling was related to. It is actually very important not to be satisfied with easing the painful feeling and to come back to the nightmare later to understand what its message is about. These messages are some of the most important ones carried by dreams.

When you come back to it a few days later, you can use any experiential method from Chapter 4 or any art therapy method from Chapter 5 to complete your dreamwork.

6
Lucid Dreaming and Awakening of Self

Saphrael and Floraniel

I am at the family farm, in the bedroom I occupied during the first 18 years of my life. Lying on my back, I feel the window behind me. I rise above the bed. As I get closer to the ceiling, weightlessness induces a sense of well-being. I stop at about 60 centimeters (24") from the ceiling and, still on my back, I head toward the window. I am thinking of the obstacle that will be coming soon, while hoping this moment to be prolonged. Then I realise that I am dreaming and I think to myself that going through the obstacle is the way to go. I feel a rush of pleasure at that thought and, once I get near the wall, I run forward. I go through the wall with such energy that I find myself hovering above the field behind the house, about ten meters (25') above the ground and several meters from my bedroom's window!

I feel the space open up all around my body and decide to turn on my stomach. I am moving ever upward. I am now more than 10 meters (25') away and I am speeding. I suddenly feel overcome by the freedom that followed my decision to go ahead. The landscape is breathtaking, and I know I am dreaming ... and that does not stop me from dreaming. My sense of ecstasy is enhanced.

I feel excited about what will follow. A mountain range appears on the horizon. It is similar to the Himalayas. Now I know I have just left my familiar world. I am at a very high altitude and yet I have the feeling to see clear details such as mountain ridges, streams, snow-capped peaks and, especially, the light in which everything is bathed.

Suddenly, I am seeing the edge of a coniferous forest in the distance, on my left. It is an overall picture of a huge expanse that seems to sit at the bottom of a large valley extending from east to west. I suddenly focus on a point on the edge of the forest. This point quickly takes on the traits of a human being who waves at me. In the blink of an eye, I stand at his side. His name is Saphrael. In his forties, he has long and tangled blond hair. In short, he looks like a hippie from the seventies and indeed wears a tunic with a floral print. Saphrael extends his arm and I now see a second character named Floraniel. They are virtually identical. I see them as brothers. Extending his arm, Saphrael points to the northwest and says, "Here is the original forest that has been here ever since the winds started blowing." I realise that the mountain range was covered with forests in the past. I now see Floraniel has gained weight; he is wearing a toga and sitting in a meditative posture.

The dream is coming to an end. At the same time, I start going backward at full speed. Saphrael and Floraniel are now two distant points and I feel on the verge of waking up. I start sobbing as after a particularly intense dream. I wake up on it. I feel deeply touched by the memories of that clear vision and the joy of meeting these two characters whom I believe to be personal guides.

Dreamer's comments

This is one of the most important dreams of my life. This is a lucid dream where I see reality with an increased sense of clarity, both in my thoughts and in my visual perception of things. Through this experience, I realise how much dreaming is in itself an aspect of reality. I had always postulated that reality was the one we are aware of in waking life and that the other one, the dream realm, was only a reflection of it. Just like a full moon on a clear night only reflects the sun rays. I now understand that they are two different states of consciousness and there is no need to subordinate one or the other. Dreams somewhat reflect our waking life because the main actor is the same in both, not because the reality of dreams is less real or less true than that of our waking life.

According to a combination of events or personal inclinations that I do not yet grasp clearly, I can access a state of consciousness during dreaming which is comparable to the one I feel at the time I am writing this, for example. However, that lucidity condition during dreams gives access to a range of potentials far exceeding the possibilities of motion, encounters or mise-en-scène that are otherwise available to me during waking life.

I am left with the impression that this experience is only the first step of a long staircase leading to ever-increasing lucidity and quality experience. The amazing sharp vision, which allowed me to see many details of the mountains and valleys while passing over the mountain range, lasted only a brief moment. How would it have been if I had become aware at the time that it was possible to get closer, see, feel and have a taste of the different features of the landscape, such as flowers, trees or streams? In this way, I would have maintained a state of consciousness similar to that of waking life where it is up to me, for example, to stop working and allow time for seeing, smelling or tasting a flower or a blade of grass, only this time in a context where the range of possibilities is commensurate with the range of my imagination.

I understand that in my dream life, dreams reflect some dynamic forces that are simply not available during waking life, through various symbols. My dreaming life will always be a faithful companion and a reflection of my psychic reality; it will provide an endless supply of insights and lessons applicable to my everyday life. But that dream helped me realise that our dreaming life goes beyond normal dreams, although the latter provide a lot of material. I may have inadvertently entered a palace and, although I forgot how to get there, I want to find my way back. The dream I have just told has opened up a fascinating inner world. The capacity to access this state of consciousness will always feel as a privilege to me.

This dream and the dreamer's comments typically illustrate the writings on lucid dreaming. They both reflect the feeling of ecstasy, the visual acuity, the enthusiastic discovery of an uncommon state of consciousness, as well as the certainty that lucid dreams irrevocably change the perception of reality, as much in one's dream life as in waking life.

Scott Sparrow talks about this phenomenon as follows: "*Yet, that which transpires during a single lucid dream may be of immeasurably greater value to the dreamer than a normal dream*" (1982, p. 23).

The Meaning of Lucid Dreaming from a Psychological Perspective

Among all the authors whose works I studied, Scott Sparrow (1992), P. Garfield (1995, 1979) and Robert Waggoner (2015, 1973) are the authors who offer the most extensive thinking on lucid dreaming, especially about the meaning of its emergence in the life of a dreamer from a psychological perspective. This section is largely inspired from them. They compare the transition from normal dreams to lucid dreaming to the emergence of ego, in other words to the emergence of self-awareness in the primitive psyche, in both primitive humans and children. Sparrow (1992) demonstrates that lucid dreaming is one step in the process of personal evolution toward consciousness or, as Jung said, in the individuation process.

Now let's take a closer look at how Sparrow describes the typical level of consciousness in a normal symbolic dream:

There is something curiously similar between the normal dream state and the consciousness of primitive man. In the dream, an individual possesses what seems to be a conscious identity, but rarely does it dawn upon the dreamer that things in the dream could be other than they are.

The dreamer does not question the necessity of the experience or what could be done to alter the circumstances. Self-reflection is rarely present in the normal dream state.

In the normal state of dreaming, an individual does not dream in the sense of it being a willed or chosen activity. Instead it is an experience which comes to him, which happens to him (1982, p. 15).

He further explains what happens during the transition from the normal dream state into lucid dreaming: The dreamer is required to establish a boundary between himself and the dream, which means he has to set himself as a separate entity from the dream's environment. Sparrow uses the Gestalt concept of contact boundary to explain this phenomenon. The dreamer is actually separating clearly his personal boundaries from the dream's boundaries, instead of being in a state of confluence with it. The state of confluence is akin to the one in a young child who cannot yet make a psychological distinction between himself and his mother, or to the one in a primitive human who do not see himself as a subject (observer) in his environment, but as an object (entity) in an environment whose influence he is under.

These explanations allow us to see the meaning of the following statement: "We dream as we live and we live as we dream." Most of the time, we see life as something that happens to us. We never question our lives, perceiving reality as immutable and being under its influence. Our awareness of what we feel is very partial, much like for most of our normal symbolic dreams. We are somehow absent from ourselves.

The onset of lucid dreaming in our lives marks a consciousness breakthrough into our usual ocean of unconsciousness. While it happens quite often to have a lucid dream almost inadvertently, it is more difficult to replicate the experience at will. For something in us desperately desires to remain unconscious.

In lucid dreaming, we are clearly conscious that our will is independent from the dream images and that we have the capacity to take action on them. Our perceptive acuity is enhanced and we can change events or our reactions to events; we also experience intense emotions and great joy in particular.

These words could just as well describe how individuals with greater self-consciousness feel: They can influence the direction of their lives; they perceive themselves as driving forces and actors across the complex web of forces that shape their lives, rather than feeling victimised by forces beyond their control or the malice of others. When we succeed in feeling that way in waking life, is there not great joy just as in lucid dreaming?

Also, we dream as we live. But since we also live as we dream, our dreaming world can be used to grow in consciousness, which will be reflected in waking life (Waggoner and McCreedy, 2015). Dreaming can be used as a laboratory where new abilities are experimented and consequently more easily reflected in waking life.

Similarly, I think that growing in consciousness in one's dream life through lucid dreaming will be reflected in waking life, thus leading to greater lucidity being experienced. One mirrors the other. Lucid dreaming marks the awakening of self-presence in waking life and provides an opportunity to further develop self-presence, to "living lucidly" (Waggoner and McCready, 2015). In this vein, here is a wonderful quote from Patricia Garfield:

Observing how we live our life is like becoming conscious that we are dreaming while dreaming. Once awaken to our emotions and to the implications of our behavior, we are able to consciously choose a direction. In waking life as well as in dreaming, our mind becomes clearer (1979).

How to Induce Lucid Dreaming

How do we achieve lucid dreaming? This is a question that is frequently addressed in the relevant literature. Among others, Stephen Laberge (2008, 1990, 1985), an expert in lucid dreaming research at Stanford University and Howard Rheingold (1990), researcher in the field of brain, creativity and cognitive functions, Gagliardi (2016) and Robert Waggoner with Carole McCready (2015) have all developed extensive knowledge about how lucid dreaming can be induced.

First of all, even for experts, lucid dreams are infrequent. So, having lucid dreams at will means having a few ones a month, which suggests a number of steps need to be taken in order to achieve this. Based on my readings, my experience and that of some of my clients and my partner, I have been able to establish four guiding principles that can help us achieve this. They are detailed as follows.

Incubation of Lucid Dreaming

Incubation is about immersing oneself in the dreaming world, by all available means. For example, you might want to read about lucid dreaming, talk about it, share with experienced people, imagine with them what it might be like, make one up in writing, or any other means that comes to mind. If you have the opportunity to take some time off in an environment free from any distractions, all the better. But such ideal conditions are not absolutely required for incubation. Reading about the matter and talking about it often have the exact same effect. Giving a lot of attention to one's dreaming life by writing a Dream Journal regularly and extensively is another easy way to immerse in your dreamworld. In short, anything that can help you connect with your dream world in general, and with lucid dreams in particular, will set the stage.

You may go to bed expressing a clear intention to have a lucid dream and give yourself a specific goal, for example flying up in the sky or going to a specific location. You need to repeat the intention to yourself many times as you go to bed. You would then be using the "the power of suggestion" (Waggoner and McCready, 2015). These authors suggest writing three sentences in your Dream Journal and then, to circle the one suggestion that appeals to you the most, rewording it if necessary to fit your taste. These three sentences are:

Tonight, in my dreams, I will realise I am dreaming and become consciously aware (or I will allow myself to ...).

Tonight, in my dreams, I will be more critically aware, and when I experience something odd, I will realise I am dreaming and become lucid (or I allow myself to be more critically aware).

Tonight in my dreams, some part of me will stay aware and then inform me when I am dreaming, so I will realise I am dreaming (e.g. the part of you that wakes you up exactly at 4 a.m. to catch an early airplane flight, even before your alarm clock rings a minute later) (Waggoner and McCready, 2015, p. 37).

Linking Waking Life to Dream States

Many techniques mentioned in the literature on lucid dreams aim to create as many links as possible between waking life and dreaming states, starting with the technique created by famous author Carlos Castaneda (1976), suggesting to look at the palm of one's hand while dreaming, and to practice looking closely at it several times a day. Gackenbach and Bosweld (1989) suggest the following version with slight differences:

> Write the letter **C** (for **C**onscience) on the palm of your hand. Every time you see it, ask yourself the following question: "Is this real or am I dreaming?" Then take a look around and deliberately test the reality of the place where you are (p. 32).

The authors suggest doing this exercise several times a day, creating opportunities to ask that same question and test reality both when asleep and while dreaming. Waggoner and McCready (2015) also suggest a slight variation from Castaneda. Basically, they suggest to look at the palm of your hand in a relaxed manner just before going to sleep and to repeat to yourself the suggestion: "Tonight while I am dreaming, I will see my hands and realise that I am dreaming" (p. 34).

According to Jean Gagliardi (2016), one of the best ways to promote lucid dreaming is to practice mindfulness meditation. He suggests proceeding as follows:

> To experience this, just start with becoming aware of your body. As you are likely sitting down: Feel the areas where your body is in touch with the seat; be mindful of tensions, if any, or feelings of discomfort or relaxation. To go one step further, be mindful of your breathing without attempting to change anything. Finally, be mindful of your inner mood: What is present? How do you feel and what thoughts come to mind? Is your mind restless? Do you have questions and/or criticisms while reading this article? Do not try to change them or direct them. Just keep on observing (2016, voiedureve.Blogspot.com/rêvelucide. Free translation).

There are other ways to promote lucid dreaming, such as reviewing the dreams noted in order to identify any opportunities favorable to lucidity, in other words potential pre-lucidity cues, which actually are gateways to lucid dreaming. Here are a few examples:

- When I am not satisfied with what happens in a dream, without becoming lucid.
- When there are incongruities in a dream, in other words events that are impossible in waking life, like being airborne, or else facts contrary to my day-to-day reality.

- When I spontaneously change the end of a dream without actually becoming aware that I am dreaming.

These opportunities for lucidity are more easily identified during dreaming when one makes a habit of writing down these missed opportunities in one's Dream Journal while awake.

There are many more ways to practice becoming lucid while dreaming. These are just the basic ones. The underlying principle of all these exercises is to try to narrow the gap between one's waking state and one's dreaming state, so that a conscious intention during daytime becomes conscious while dreaming; in other words, daytime consciousness enters nighttime consciousness. On the other hand, it seems that the opposite, that is, seeking to bring one's dream life into one's waking life as much as possible, is just as effective. For example, if a situation occurring during the day reminds you of a dream, you should dwell on it specifically, take the time to remember it and let any other dreams that arise come back to memory. In this way, you can come to remember a whole series of similar dreams spread over several months, even those you did not take note of. These are all means to narrow the artificial gap between the waking state and the dream state.

Finally, reproducing symbols or parts of a dream through artwork is a great way to cause these two realities to intermingle. Giving a concrete form to dream images automatically causes them to come to existence. Such a powerful exercise enhances the transformative power of symbols. Methods to replicate dream symbols through art are found in Chapter 5.

Overcoming Fears and Resistances to Lucid Dreaming

Although the desire to have lucid dreams is very present at times, it is not always enough to access this type of experience. Something in us demonstrates a strong resistance to ascend into higher consciousness and to leave the protective matrix of the unconscious mind. Aside from this basic resistance, Scott Sparrow (1982) makes it very clear that experiencing inner conflicts, which we all experience, forms barriers between the unconscious mind, where such conflicts lie, and the inherent ability of each individual to have lucid dreams. Therefore, the first step to be taken toward deliberate lucid dreaming is to work on one's inner conflicts. Your ordinary dreams offer a wealth of information about these types of conflicts and the methods to work on your symbolic dreams can therefore increase the permeability, a term used by Scott Sparrow:

> *Although capacity [to have lucid dreams] is potentially available, it becomes accessible only to the degree that an individual is permeable, or relatively free of unreconciled conflicts which form barriers. When a person is permeable, desire [to have lucid dreams] then stimulates or invites the influx of capacity into conscious awareness. This process may culminate in a healing dream or a deep meditative experience in which a*

union occurs between the conscious, aspiring individual and the deeper, transforming self (1982, p. 28).

In other words, although initial lucid dreams may arise spontaneously, and even without any conscious desire to experience that, experiencing deliberate lucid dreams is more likely to happen after undertaking or pursuing a personal growth process.

Furthermore, any excessive desire to have lucid dreams may also hinder access to that experience. When internal conflicts are relatively resolved, one must be willing to let go of the ego desire to control and be humble enough to wait. For example, the day I thought to myself that it was pointless, that I had no capacity for lucid dreaming, I had a dream where I experienced a lucid state for a few seconds. I called that dream *The Crack in the Cosmic Egg*, inspired by the name of the book (Pearce, 2002).

The belief that you have no capacity for lucid dreaming might be an obstacle that needs to be worked on. Research by Gackenbach & Bosweld (1989) demonstrates that most people can learn to have lucid dreams; they also state that 58% of the population have at least one spontaneous lucid dream in their lifetime.

Through my dream *The Crack in the Cosmic Egg*, I became aware of some blockages within myself. During the few seconds I experienced lucidity, I entered a tunnel filled with wonderful colors and shapes. I recognised the magic land of my youth that I was visiting at will every night. The memory of this magic land came back while reading a book from Joyce Petschek (1982), an artist and speaker about Tibetan Buddhist spirituality, in which a similar land was described. I had totally forgotten about that experience! I remembered that by the age of twelve, I had felt very sad the day I became aware that I could no longer access this wonderland at will. I promised myself that I would go back some day.

Through this dream, I discovered that lucid dreaming could be a wonderful, beautiful and magical experience, instead of a painful one where I must be able to stay on track and keep myself from "lower fringe demons" as suggested by Patricia Garfield (1979). These were my unconscious fears about lucid dreaming. No, thank you! I did not want anything to do with them and I did not have a clue about what to do if I ever met them! I must admit I just did not feel strong enough to face my own personal demons. After discovering through this first dream that lucid dreaming can be an ecstatic experience, I found the experience more inviting and I had fewer objections.

In some ways, having a lucid dream is like dying – dying to our habitual perception of things and to the control of our ego on the conscious world. This is likely another unconscious objection. Whenever there is a major change in our personal level of awareness, there comes a time when we actually feel we are dying, and that fear feels real. To some extent, thus, the ego must also be ready to die to itself.

Various means are available to identify your fears and blockages concerning lucid dreams. They are the following:

- You may share your fears and your reluctance with friends who are also interested in the matter.
- You may read authors who write about lucid dreaming experiences. Their writings may potentially help you identify any fears and any reluctance you have. See Waggoner and McCready (2015) and Kelzer (1990) in particular.
- You can ask to get answers from your dreams. In other words, ask for an incubation dream to learn about what prevents you from having lucid dreams, then work on this dream the following day, whatever it is.
- You can also do the following exercise. Please write down "I do not want to have lucid dreams because …", then complete the sentence by stating all the "reasons why" coming spontaneously to mind, even if they seem far-fetched, utterly irrational or that you do not understand them at first; avoid too much thinking and censoring. The outcomes will come as a surprise, and you will likely realise in what you wrote down that your objections are about one or two key reasons. You will then have brought out one or more of your fears and/or your reluctance or objections. When brought to consciousness, fears diminish and potentially their power over you lessens. Any objection that has become conscious can be evaluated and then set aside. Repeat the exercise regularly to bring out any opposition, until you successfully have lucid dreams. This exercise alone is not necessarily enough to experience lucid dreaming, but it has the same role as incubation, which is to set the stage for it. Here is an example:

"I do not want to have lucid dreams because …"

- I am afraid of the intense feelings and even more of the joy I might experience (well, well, what a surprise!)
- I will have to deal with the unknown
- It is too good to be true
- I am afraid to change
- I am afraid of feeling sadness when rediscovering the lost world of my childhood

The last sentence sounded especially right, just like the first that came to my mind about being afraid of intense feelings whether it be joy or sorrow. No deep thinking was needed to become aware of the current blockage: The fear of intense feelings, at the time. Writing extensively is often needed to identify barriers. So, do not be upset if you find yourself filling out a whole page.

Looking for Gratification in Dreams

Indeed, as it seems that lucid dreams often generate a sense of satisfaction and intense pleasure, the search for pleasure in ordinary dreams achieves closer access to lucid dreaming. I think this is why Patricia Garfield (1995) considers the incubation of a dream of flight as a preparatory stage to lucid dreaming. In addition, she thinks that lucid dreamers have more frequent dreams of flying than ordinary dreamers. Along the same lines, the Senoi people/tribe from Malaysia, who daily used dreams and systematically developed their lucid dreaming skills, suggested to always head toward orgasm in dreams of a sexual nature (Morris, 2002).

Therapeutic Use of Lucid Dreaming

Lucid dreaming often portrays unexplored parts of us, extraordinary potentials to actualise as well as good opportunities for personal growth. In addition, we are often confronted with non-integrated or conflicting parts. Since we are aware that we are dreaming, lucid dreams can be used to work on the integration of polarities or unconscious parts. Here are different ways to use them for therapeutic purposes:

- Initiating a dialogue with a character from a lucid dream, especially if it is an individual who first appears as an enemy, in an attempt to get to know him and to reconcile with him;
- Actually getting into the character's body, a powerful lucid dreaming way to practice Gestalt identification;
- Acting in a way that is assertive and non-aggressive in order to resolve a situation. The confidence experienced when you successfully solve a problem while dreaming seems to transfer into waking life.

In fact, dreamwork methods used for usual symbolic dreams can be used for lucid dreaming as if you were doing dreamwork as the dream unfolds.

In the end, working on ordinary dreams and seeking to have lucid dreams often allow the same goals to be achieved, that is, greater self-consciousness. Although lucid dreaming is a step forward in your personal evolution, it does not devalue symbolic dreams as a source of growth. The following example accurately illustrates how work on lucid dreaming and symbolic dreams both generate awareness.

Example of a symbolic dream followed with a lucid dream

The following dreams were shared by one of my clients:

The Plowed Fields

I am in the countryside in plowed fields. It is springtime. A combined harvester-thresher goes downhill quite slowly and there is nobody on board.

I am frozen in surprise, there is no time to escape! So, I decide to lie down on the ground, hoping the combined harvester-thresher will pass overhead without causing injuries.

How wrong I was! As the harvester passes, the metal teeth graze my legs. The harvester continues slowly downhill. My injured legs are killing me and I have trouble walking.

The dreamer got up because her baby was crying. She asked to get clarity in her next dream because she did not get the message. Then she had the following dream.

> *I am in the same fields and they have to be plowed. My sister and her boyfriend tell me the process, since I know nothing about it. Hand in hand, they are on their way in order to plow the neighboring fields. I have to start with a small area of about three meters. The machinery is gigantic. I do not see how I can make a fairly good job in such a small area. Why are they insisting on that stretch of land, moreover downhill, whereas the fields are extensive, large and flat?*
>
> *I get into the tractor, despite my injured and sore legs. Taking the wheel, I start the engine; brakes are broken or almost inoperative. I am pumping the brakes again and again, then I wake up, feeling frightened.*

Since she still did not understand these painful and difficult images, she reiterated her request for clarification. Then the dream became a lucid one.

The Accident

> *I see a crowd gathered at the scene of a motor accident. I am one of three victims; the other two are my brother and my sister. This is a motor accident in a side street, at the intersection of a busy street, maybe in Montreal!*
>
> *I am in an "astral" plane, looking for my body. I then see my mother running to the accident site. She seems distraught to see the damage. Cars are nothing more than a pile of twisted wrecks. The paramedics rush to get the wounded out of the cars. My body seems to be the most messed up of the three. People fear that I will not survive.*
>
> *I call out to my mother and ask her if she knows where my body is. She tells me that my body has virtually been broken to pieces and that my sister and my brother are badly injured; then she tells me where my body is.*
>
> *The situation seems absurd, totally unacceptable and unthinkable. I consciously decide not to reintegrate my injured body. I refuse to suffer! I am moving straight ahead in a troubled street. My mother feels proud of me and encourages me to move along that way.*

This person chose to do dreamwork in a group. She was at a point in her life where all sorts of unexpected and sudden changes were happening, like losing her job and the need to move out in a short period of time. Also, she felt cornered as though she had to relocate some heavy equipment. By looking at her dream, she understood that she could choose not to be overwhelmed by the situation and find ways to give herself more time to react, instead of feeling paralyzed by fear, as in the dream. For example, she could explore options with her landlord, for she suddenly remembered that she was offered to occupy the house for the summer if she so wished. Consequently, she suddenly saw herself as capable of actions, rather than as a helpless victim.

The existential message is to avoid the path of needless suffering. In fact, she may indeed journey on joyfully and quite easily by taking care of herself, rather than experiencing pain. It is interesting to note that through lucid dreaming, in response to her request for clarifications, she was presented with a similar situation where she made the conscious decision to avoid suffering. This case shows that lucid dreams and symbolic dreams both generate awareness, since they both offer opportunities to work on the same inner process. Referring to this, Scott Sparrow (1992) argues that the process of taking responsibility for the dream through lucidity gets very close to the purpose of the Gestalt approach, which is of developing self-awareness.

Such a lucid dream needs further discussion. We could indeed question the relevance of "leaving the body behind", avoiding pain and personal growth process. Many searchers about lucid dreaming warn dreamers against the tendency to use lucid dreams for the purpose of avoiding unpleasant situations, it then becomes some means to avoid journeying rather than a way to cope with one's inner conflicts. In the present instance, though, I do not think it would have been a wise decision to reintegrate a body that was in such a bad shape, although symbolically. The first step is actually to choose to live something other than needless suffering and thus to take responsibility for one's future. In addition, the choice to take care of herself to avoid experiencing so much suffering will eventually help her cope with the initial suffering that resulted in leaving her body behind.

Being Mindful of Lucid Dreaming – a Word of Caution

All of that points out an important aspect of the therapeutic use of lucid dreaming. Many searchers, including Robert Waggoner and Carole McCready (2015), Scott Sparrow (1992), Kenneth Kelzer (1990) and Ann Faraday (1997), stress the importance of not trying to control lucid dreams. Trying to control dreams would mean, among other things, deciding what will be experienced, the places to visit and the persons to meet. Experts in the field rather suggest to attempt to test ways to respond in an efficient and satisfactory manner to what occurs in a dream or even to ask for information beyond your conscious knowledge with an "unlimited intent" (Waggoner and McCready, 2015). Thus, dreaming becomes an opportunity for learning and self-discovery.

Ensuring that our dreams always have a happy ending is sometimes a way to avoid facing our fears; this is not making maximum use of the possibilities of lucid dreaming. After all, as Sparrow says, the goal is to be reconciled with the elements of a dream, instead of trying to control it. It is through this lack of control, he argues, that we may actually access enlightenment (1982). Indeed, lucid dreams allow to access new powers and a new freedom, and invite us subsequently to surrender to the experience. At that moment, the ecstasy of enlightenment occurs, that is to say, the precious moment sought after in every meditation process: A connection with the sacred.

In the conclusion section, we will go back to the word "enlightenment" and its meaning. For now, let's say that lucid dreaming is experimenting self-presence, a higher state of consciousness. Over time, this ability may possibly transfer to waking life.

7
Process Dreamwork: A One-Month Intensive Dreamwork

Developing one's own dreamwork style and following one's personal process are two ways to delve even further into the personal growth approach through dreaming.

Once you are familiar with the methods, the next step is to create your own way of experiencing dreams, one that totally suits you. It is about identifying your preferred methods and those that give the most satisfying results as well as ensuring self-pacing.

The intensive one-month approach outlined in the next pages aims at learning quite quickly about the dreaming world and the various dreamwork approaches. Specifically, the objectives of the suggested approach are the following.

- To integrate your Dream Journal and your dreamworking practice into waking life.
- To get familiar with as many methods as possible in order to identify the most suitable ones for you.

The suggested approach is designed to move forward in a way that facilitates learning about the methods. However, you may also want to plan your own intensive one-month process; it will prove to be effective to the extent that it is tailored to your preferences and needs and allows for experimenting as many methods as possible.

Finding One's Own Pace

An intensive one-month process helps fully embrace your dreamworld. At first, constant effort is needed to keep your focus on the dream world and to become familiar with the images and symbols it carries. As dreamwork will have been made a habit after this intensive period, your pace will get settled; it will probably decrease significantly after this first month. Dreamwork should always be fun; it is not about forcing yourself to keep a Dream Journal and then feeling guilty when you take a break.

The intensive process described below requires a substantial time investment as well as a significant emotional commitment given it will likely trigger an intensive inner transformation process. If you prefer to modulate the pace to proceed much more slowly, just stage the process over a longer stretch of time. The process suggested below should require about 45 minutes a day in the first week, one to two hours a day in the second and third weeks, and three two-hour periods in the last week.

Week 1:   Write in your *Dream Journal*. I recommend trying a different Creative writing method every day (See Chapter 3).

Week 2:   Write in your *Dream Journal*. Practice the identification method or the Gestalt dialogue approach every day (See Chapter 4).

Week 3:   Write in your *Dream Journal*. Practice one of the three other experiential methods every day: The Jungian dialogue approach, Exploring the sounds and movements or Re-entry into a dream (see Chapter 4).

Week 4:   Write in your *Dream Journal*. Practice one of the art therapy methods three times a week: Drawing, Three-dimensional reproduction of a dream, Drawing the elusive sensation from a dream or Draw a quick sketch to appease a nightmare (See Chapter 5).

Description of the Intensive Process

Writing in one's *Dream Journal* obviously forms the basis for any dreamwork. Indeed, as mentioned in Chapter 2, the mere act of writing down dreams raises self-awareness. Such self-awareness in waking life helps becoming aware over time of our inner reactions to people and events, instead of living in limbo, without knowing what is going on in our inner world. Jotting down our dreams on paper automatically triggers a self-awareness process. You might want to make a habit of keeping your *Dream Journal*, even when you are not doing dreamwork; that is why the writing step will remain as a systematic instruction during the four weeks.

For the first week, just use the creative writing methods. Try to use various ones to experiment as many as possible, in order to broaden your own repertoire. Your favorite ones will be easily identified; nevertheless, keep in mind that the goal is to become familiar with all of them. Specific conditions are attached to the programming methods used to change recurrent dreams and for incubation dreams, as they might involve repetition several nights in a row, possibly for weeks. So, you may try them to ensure you understand, knowing they might not give immediate results.

The second week is about learning the basic Gestalt methods. More than any others, these ultimate experiential methods enable to gain a better understanding of how dreams reflect one's life experience and refer primarily to oneself. I think that this is what is basically learned from dreamwork.

The third week, it is suggested that you become familiar with the other experiential methods – in other words the *Jungian dialogue approach*, *Exploring the sounds and movements of a dream* or *Re-entry into a dream* – always for the purpose of identifying the ones that actually suit you and broadening your own repertoire.

Finally, the fourth week is for learning about art therapy methods. About two hours will be required to experiment each method. Make sure to purchase in advance any art materials you might need.

Following One's Process

It is important to familiarise yourself with several methods for various reasons. Of course, you will enjoy a few ones more than others. In addition, some are better suited for certain types of dreams. Nevertheless, it will be of even greater benefit for your personal dreamwork process if you use several of them consecutively. Arnol Mindell (1985), a Jungian analyst, and Joseph Goodbread (1987), a psychologist, developed an approach called process-oriented psychology, that will be applied to dreams below. Alexandra Duchastel (2005) also explained the process-oriented approach in her book on art therapy.

The process-oriented approach requires using several methods to explore a single dream. To do so, you need to be mindful of what is going on inside of you as you go along. I consider this approach as an advanced method, to be used only after many months of dreamwork, because it requires a broad experience in terms of in-depth dreamwork. Being familiar with self-work for personal growth can also be of great help. This is my preferred method because it is highly flexible in use. In other words, I value all the methods mentioned in this book, as long as they are suitable for one's immediate inner experience. Their relevance in relation to one's own experience is the overriding criterion.

Since it closely tracks the deployment of one's inner experience, this method makes it possible to get more directly to the core of the issue, like an arrow reaching the center of a target. It is better to be familiar with self-work before undertaking this.

The following example illustrates how process-oriented psychology can be applied to dreams:

- As an example, I undertake dreamwork using the Gestalt identification method;
- Then I proceed with the Jungian dialogue, as I often do, in order to gain a better understanding of the involvement of a particular character in my dream;
- While dialoguing with this character, a vague and unclear feeling raises, then I focus on it by using the meditation on the elusive sensation;
- Just as I focus on this vague and elusive sensation, an image pops up from my imagination. I make a drawing of it;

- After drawing, I write about any associations and feelings that this image brings up, and the existential message then becomes clear. The last step is to find any practical applications for my waking life.

This self-work method based on dreams makes it possible to elucidate the existential message of the dream in a nuanced way. It actually is a real self-exploration and autotherapy session. It also clearly implies a significant and fascinating emotional experience generating inner transformations; therefore, going through such a profound experience requires a certain time commitment. To help you understand what it means to follow one's process, I developed a few points of reference that will be proposed below.

I believe in the humanist postulate of organismic wisdom in every human being, a wisdom that seeks to manifest itself whenever it is given the opportunity. The process is simply the path followed by our experience to produce the inner transformation required for our greatest self-fulfillment.

Following your process is about paying attention to everything that is spontaneously brought up during dreamwork, because these are clues about the process seeking to deploy. When focusing on a dream, the following can be brought up:

- Physical sensations;
- Pain or body tension;
- Specific feelings;
- Images or symbols;
- Spontaneous inner dialogue;
- Intuitions and ideas.

This method requires to pay attention to these clues and to use them as points of reference in order to select the most appropriate dreamwork method as you go along, the one allowing to amplify them and thus be able to decode the dream's existential message. The following are examples of typical clues and appropriate methods for amplification:

Clues from an Ongoing Process	Possible Appropriate Methods
Physical Sensations	
• Vague or elusive sensations • Involuntary movements • Feeling like moving body parts • Any other physical sensation	• Meditation on the elusive sensation • Exploring the sounds and movements from the dream • Drawing the movements • Painting the physical sensation

Clues from an Ongoing Process	Possible Appropriate Methods
Body Pain and Tension	
• Back pain, headache, nauseas, etc.	• Drawing the dream • Drawing the pain • Meditation on the pain or tension, same as meditating on the elusive sensation
Specific Feelings	
• Sorrow, anger, joy, love, tenderness, disgust, resentment, fear, etc.	• Drawing or painting the key feeling from the dream • Exploring the dream's sounds and movements associated with emotions (crying, sounds of joy, etc.)
Images or Symbols	
• Spontaneous images, specific dream images, old memories	• Drawing or painting images • Three-dimensional reproduction of images or symbols • Gestalt identification • Spontaneous associations • Heuristic map • Re-entry into a dream
Spontaneous Inner Dialogue	
• Any imaginary inner dialogue with oneself or someone else • Feeling like having a conversation with an intriguing character or object from the dream	• Gestalt dialogue • Jungian dialogue
Intuitions or Ideas	
• Intuitions or ideas about the dream's existential message (Intuitions and ideas are helpful when the experiential work actually took place and when used to clearly state the message to remember)	• A heuristic map of all intuitions or ideas associated with the dream and the existential message • A clear statement about the existential message and the practical applications

Example of dreamwork using the process-oriented approach

The following dream is from the person who had the series of dreams about snakes shared in Chapter 1.

The Pearly Shell

As I bend down, I see a small hole in the ground that looks like a shell. I notice there is no water in it and this detail seems important, as I expected there would be. The sun reflects against the inner layers of the shell even if there is no water. The salmon-colored inner layers look like flesh. (See Figure 7.1.)

Here are the steps followed by the dreamer for the dreamwork:

She undertakes the Gestalt identification process in order to explore the shell image:

I am a shell without water. The sun warms my inner layers. These are pearly, flesh-colored and pinkish beige. I am beautiful and soft. I lay on the ground.

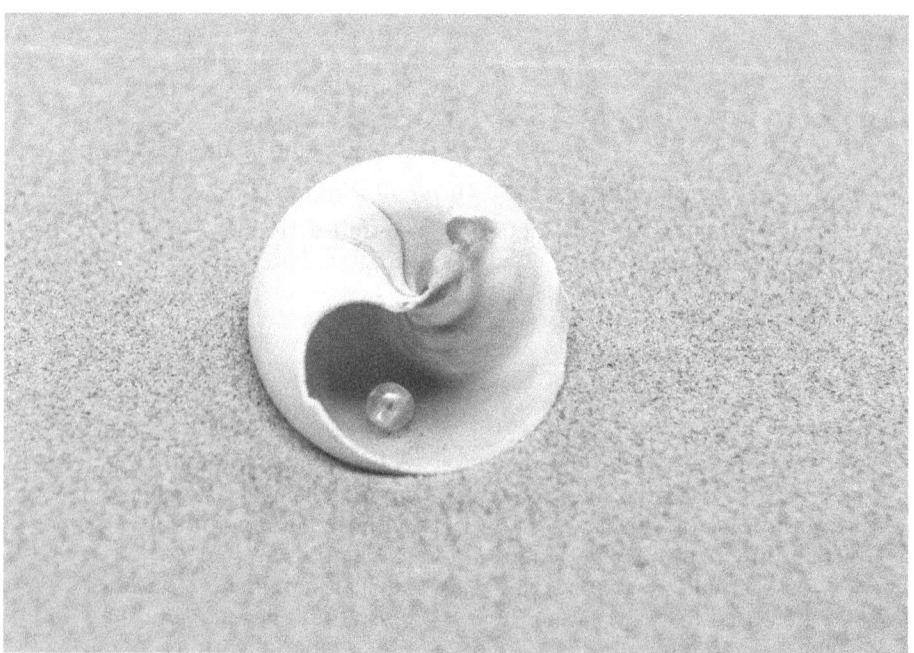

Figure 7.1 *The Pearly Shell.* Shell, pearl and sand. Photograph Credit: Michelle Boulay, Sherbrooke, Qc. Canada.

She goes on with the Jungian dialogue since she finds intriguing the presence of the shell in the dream and feels like asking questions.

Dreamer:	*Why is it important for you to have water or not?*
Shell:	*When I have water, I also have a pearl!*
Dreamer:	*What does the water represent thus?*
Shell:	*Water is the source of life; water is fertile and filled with potential life. There is no water in the shell, you are just imagining there is.*
Dreamer:	*And what about you, what do you represent, pearl?*
Pearl:	*I am the crowning of life, the gift of life and the gift that comes with water; I show up when there is water. In this dream, I almost go unnoticed, because there is no water in the shell. To see me, you have to imagine there is water in the shell.*

At this point, the dreamer starts to relate the pearl and water to pregnancy. Since the existential message has not yet emerged clearly, she decides to go on with the three-dimensional reproduction of the dream. She uses the shell image that asserts itself in her imagination as the primordial image of the dream. See Figure 7.1: The shell on the ground is reproduced in a sandplay box. Then she writes about her reactions and spontaneous associations with the object that was created:

There is actually water in the shell and it feels good. The shell becomes heavy when I add water, which confirms to me that water symbolises pregnancy in the present instance. I add a pearl and I find it really quite beautiful. However, in my dream, there is no water. So, I decide to remove the water to feel the difference it makes. Without water, the pearly inner layers of the shell are more apparent and it is also magnificent. It's a different kind of beauty, but it's no less beautiful. The sun is the intensity of love that feels warm, penetrates and keeps my inner layers warm!

A glimmer of insight leads to stating the dream's existential message:

The existential message has now become clear to me: The sun will warm me up even if I am not pregnant. In other words, sexuality is beautiful even outside of reproduction. I end up realising that I am still affected by the Catholic morality which considers that sexuality is only acceptable for reproduction! So, tensions associated with sexuality and pleasure still stayed with me in relation to that. I can hardly believe that this idea, long since rejected, still influenced me. Indeed, the prohibitions against sexual pleasure are very tenacious in my society!

Finally, the dreamer decides to change her beliefs:

"I never want to feel guilty again about sexuality and pleasure."

Therefore, using successive methods that stuck closely to her life experience and inner images, the dreamer was able to understand the dream's profound message. She confirmed that this experience has had profound and actual impacts on her sexuality: She experienced less tension in her sexual life and less guilt over sexual pleasure.

Conclusion

After 45 years of my own dreamwork, I can say from hindsight that I had great breakthroughs about myself and the impact of my personal story on my life. Important events in my childhood, that I had forgotten or did not know about, were brought back through dreamwork and art therapy, and this resulted in achieving greater self-awareness. The impact of this work on my life is very significant. I also believe I could not feel that happy without my exploration work from deep within!

Work on oneself is a never-ending task. We are constantly growing. Although we may feel at times that some step is coming full circle, there is always another process beginning to emerge or to develop. We dream of death and rebirth, but we never reach perfection once and for all! However, some states of well-being are fully achievable, and we can get to feel more and more fulfillment and happiness!

In concrete terms, dreamwork allows to achieve the following results:

- Achieving greater self-consciousness and awareness of one's inner world;
- Solving problems;
- Solving inner conflicts;
- Developing one's creativity;
- Gaining more control over one's behavior;
- Creating more harmonious human relationships;
- Removing unconscious barriers to one's sexuality;
- Identifying unconscious needs;
- Discovering unimagined personal potentials;
- Identifying methods for psychological and physical healing;
- Enabling psychological and spiritual growth;
- Accessing paranormal information (premonitory, clairvoyant or telepathic);
- Achieving higher states of consciousness.

From these outcomes, is it possible to portray an individual who has been doing dreamwork for a long time? I mentioned throughout this book that dreamwork helps achieve greater self-awareness. This comes down to four specific aspects, as follows.

A More Fulfilled Individual

An individual with greater self-awareness is a more fulfilled person, in other words more and more free from inner conflicts. Fulfillment is not a definitive state; it is a continuous development process. We have seen how dreams often bring out inner conflicts; now the Gestalt dialogue approach is specifically aimed at giving the opportunity to work toward resolving such conflicts. Freeing oneself from inner conflicts restores the energy previously used to struggle with one's conflicts; then it becomes available for other purposes, for example to realise one's potential and creativity.

Although inner conflicts will never cease to arise, you will first solve the most urgent ones, the most paralyzing ones for you, with the result that you will have greater energy with time.

A Proactive Individual

An individual with greater self-awareness develops a *proactive* attitude. Stephen R. Covey (2013/1989), author of several publications about leadership, was the first to use this word; he addresses seven lifestyle habits of highly efficient people. The proactive attitude is the first one of these. Here is his definition:

> *It means more than merely taking initiative. It means that as human beings, we are responsible for our own lives. Our behavior is a function of our decisions, not our conditions* (1989, p. 71).

As Stephen R. Covey so aptly says, it is not what happens to us that causes suffering, but our response to what happens to us. A proactive individual does not depend on favorable conditions in his life to feel good; he is able to reflect and decide about the most appropriate attitude to a situation, knowing that he is responsible for his well-being.

I think this is why we must seek to achieve better self-knowledge, to identify our deepest emotional experience in dealing with the circumstances and the people in our lives. Only then can we actually choose how to respond, how to adapt to life circumstances. And self-knowledge is precisely accessible through dreams. By doing dreamwork on several dreams mentioned in this book, the dreamers were able to adopt a proactive attitude. Here are a few examples:

- *Dream series about snakes* (Chapter 1)

This series of dreams ended with empowerment (the word came to mind in the dreamer's last dream); she then felt more and more able to take action in order to satisfy her emotional needs. She saw herself as more responsible for her own needs and she felt that she had more power over reality.

- *Liberating nightmare* (Chapter 3)

The dreamer decided to rewrite her dream in order to transform powerlessness, fear and inhibition of action into victory. She successfully attained a change of level, and felt her breathing changed following her efforts to have more control. This dreamwork was a turning point in her personal growth process.

- *The pearly shell* (Chapter 7)

Here, the dreamer freed herself from introjected values about sexual pleasure. An introjected value is one that is passed on by our culture and that we bought without even realising it. We are not aware of its influence. With the realisation that this value had stayed with her, the dreamer was able to determine her personal values with respect to sexuality. She decided that sexuality was beautiful and good even outside of reproduction, and to stop feeling guilty about it and about pleasure.

A Lucid and Courageous Individual

Personal growth and dreamwork does not guarantee only happy moments! Through this work, one will often face times of depression, sadness, discouragement, mourning or helplessness. Personal growth requires courage and is not just glorious! This does not preclude from greater fulfillment overall. As one of my colleague art therapists and friend, Mrs. Lorraine Dumont once told me:

> *While top people in the psychology field had a lot of fun with self-work, learned a lot about themselves and humanity, and had a richer life, their life was not necessarily easier. However, they have gained more power and lucidity over life, and in particular their lives.*

Robert Johnson (2009) talks about the inherent loneliness associated with walking one's own path, often a solitary journey given its uniqueness:

> *Ultimately every road is a Via Dolorosa, for it leads us into the issues and conflicts that every person must pass through, sometimes painfully and with heroic spirit, sometimes with sacrifice, in order to be initiated into the realm of consciousness.*
>
> *For each of us, that path is a solitary one, for we must ultimately walk it alone. No one else can tell us which final direction it should take, and no one else can walk it for us* (p. 188).

Achieving Higher States of Consciousness

People who do self-work through dreamwork provide themselves with an opportunity to reach altered states of consciousness. Now let us define what these consist of. Charles T. Tart (2001/1986) distinguishes four levels of consciousness based on a progression from fragmentation to integration (or unification, a term he precisely used).

1st level: Sleep and ordinary dreams (ordinary, not lucid);
2nd level: Normal waking consciousness;
3rd level: Genuine self-consciousness;
4th level: Objective consciousness.

Only the last two levels fall into the category of higher states of consciousness. Within the genuine self-consciousness, there is a constant self-awareness (what Tart also refers to as *self-remembering*) while being very present to what is going on around us. This state is difficult to maintain and takes a lot of practice. Here is how he defines it:

> *We would be genuinely self-conscious of our actions and internal states, see the world clearly (...), comprehend our essence desires, and have true will to do what we wish. We are finally one. We can genuinely say "I am," for there is a real self there that is far more alive and important than the passing identity states of consensus trance* (1989, p. 214).

To reach genuine self-consciousness, the author suggests two exercises: Self-observation and self-remembering. Reading his description of the exercises, I see clearly that dreamwork through experiential and art methods, especially following one's process with art, are forms of self-observation in the sense meant by this author. Moreover, lucid dreaming is a pure and simple exercise of recollection of oneself during dream states.

I believe lucid dreaming is so very exciting because for a while, we are precisely in the higher state of genuine self-consciousness that can possibly be reached on an ongoing basis during waking life. The definition quoted above tends to confirm this hypothesis. Isn't it similar to the description of lucid dreaming, where one simultaneously experiences a clear perception of the environment and of oneself?

Dreamwork is somehow equivalent to the exercises suggested by Tart to attain genuine self-consciousness. By contributing significantly to the attainment of this genuine self-consciousness, dreamwork also promotes access to the fourth level: The objective consciousness.

This fourth level is what is referred to as enlightenment by most of the authors. Tart refuses to define precisely what objective consciousness is, because he feels it cannot be described in the language of normal consciousness. Nonetheless, he quotes Gurdjieff, the spiritualist leader, who describes the fourth consciousness level as a state allowing to see things as they are, rather than as what our culture has taught us to see.

Well, this comes full circle for me! This book started with the dream about the *Clown in the mirror*. The clown invited me to follow him and to come and see beyond the looking glass ... I found this image totally fascinating, but I could not put a word on what I was invited to, other than to dare walking my own unique path. I now understand that he was inviting me to look beyond appearances, to look at the other side in order to see reality as it is, which ultimately comes up to achieve objective consciousness.

Bibliography

Barrett, D. (1992). Through a glass darkly: Images of the dead in dreams. *Omega*, 24(2), 97–108.

Baylor, G. W. & Deslauriers, D. (1987). *Le rêve, sa nature, sa fonction et une méthode d'analyse*. Sillery: Université du Québec.

Boa, F. (1994). *The Way of the dream: Conversations on Jungian dream interpretation with Marie-Louise von Franz*. Boston and London: Shambhala.

Bosnak, R. (1988). *A little course in dreams*. Boston: Shambhala.

Bosnak, R. (1992). *Pouvoir analyser ses rêves*. Montréal: Le jour.

Bosnak, R. (2007). *Embodiment. Creative imagination in medicine, art and travel*. New York: Routledge.

Buckner, B. B. (2012). *Dream yourself into being*. Lavergne, Tennessee: Blue Feather Press.

Buzan, T. & Buzan, B. (2008/1996). *Mind map book*. New York: Penguin.

Bulkeley, K. (2000). *Transforming dreams: Learning spiritual lessons from the dreams you never forget*. New York: John Wiley and Sons.

Bulkeley, K. & Bulkley, P. (2005). *Dreaming beyond death. A guide to pre-death dreams and visions*. Boston: Beacon Press.

Campbell, J. (1968). *The hero with a thousand faces*. Princeton: Princeton University Press.

Campbell, J. (1988). *The power of myth*. New York: Doubleday.

Campbell, J. (1989). *Historical atlas of world mythology. The way of the animal powers, 1; The way of the seeded earth, 11*. New York: Harper and Row.

Castaneda, C. (1976). *Journey to Ixtlan. The lessons of Don Juan*. Markham, On: Pocket Books. 8th printing.

Chevalier, J. & Gheerbrant, A. (1998). *Dictionnaire des symboles*. Paris: Robert Laffont/Jupiter.

Collectif de l'arc-en-ciel (1991). *Et si les rêves servaient à nous éveiller?* Montréal: Les Éditions Quebecor.

Corrière, R. & Hart, J. (2014). *Les Maîtres-Rêveurs. Réapprenez à vivre avec vos rêves et vos sentiments*. Kindle Edition.

Covey, S. R. (2013/1989). *The 7 habits of highly effective people. Powerful lessons in personal change. Special edition*. New York: Simon and Schuster.

Davis, J. L. & Wright, D. C. (2007). Randomized clinical trial for treatment of chronic nightmares in trauma-exposed adults. *Journal of Traumatic Stress*, 20(2), 123–133.

Dee, N. (1989). *The Dreamer's workbook*. Wellingborough, England: Aquarian Press.

Delaney, G. (1996). *Living your dreams. The classic bestseller on becoming your own dream expert*. New York: HarperCollins.

Delaney, G. (1995). *The dream kit: An all-in-one toolkit for understanding your dreams*. New York: Harper One.

Delaney, G. (1991). *Breakthrough dreaming. How to tap the power of your 24-hour mind*. New York: Bantam Book.

Desjarlais, R. R. (1991). Dreams, divination, and Yolmo ways of knowing. *Dreaming Journal of the Association for the Study of Dreams*, 1(3), 211–224.

Domhoff, W. (1985). *The mystique of dreams. A search for utopia through senoi dream theory*. Berkeley: University of California.

Duchastel, A. (2005). *La voie de l'imaginaire: Le processus en art-thérapie*. Montréal: Quebecor.

Faraday, A. (1997/1973). *Dream power*. New York: Berkley Medallion Books.

Faraday, A. (1997). *The dream game*. New York: Harper and Row.

Foreman, E. (1988). *Awakening. A Dream Journal*. New York: Tabori and Chang.

Freud, S. (2016/1900). *L'interprétation des rêves. Les fiches de lecture d'Universalis*. Kindle Ed.

Frost, S. B. (2010). *SoulCollage Evolving. An intuitive collage process for self-discovery and community*. Santa Cruz: Hanford Mead.

Gackenbach, J. & Bosveld, J. (1989). Take control of your dreams. *Psychology Today*. 27–32.

Gackenbach, J. & Bosveld, J. (2014). *Take control of your dreams: How lucid dreaming can help you uncover your hidden fears & explore the frontiers of human consciousness*. Kindle Edition.

Gagliardi, J. (2016). *La voie du rêve. Résumé d'une conférence. International Association for the Study of Dreams (IASD)*, Montréal, May 7, 2016. Http://voiedureve.blogspot.com

Garfield, P. (1979). *Pathway to ecstasy*. New York: Holt, Rhinehart and Winston.

Garfield, P. (1987). *Your child's dreams*. New York: Ballantine Books.

Garfield, P. (1988). *Women's bodies. Women's dreams*. New York: Ballantine Books.

Garfield, P. (1991). *The healing power of dreams*. New York: Simon and Schuster.

Garfield, P. (1994). *Creative dreaming. Plan and control your dreams to develop creativity, overcome fears, solve problems and create a better self* (2nd ed.). New York: Simon and Schuster.

Garfield, P. (1997). *The dream messenger: How dreams of the departed bring healing gifts*. New York: Simon and Schuster.

Gendlin, E. T. (1998). *Focusing Oriented Psychotherapy*. New York: Guilford Press.

Gendlin, E. T. (2011). *Let your body interpret your dreams*. Wilmette, IL.: Chiron.

Ginger, S. (2003). *La gestalt, une thérapie de contact*. Paris: Homme set groupes. 7th edition.

Godard, M. O. (2003). *Rêves et traumatismes ou la longue nuit des rescapés*. Ramonville Saint-Agen: Érès.

Goodbread, J. H. (1987). *The dreambody toolkit. A practical introduction to the philosophy, goals and practice of process-oriented psychology.* New York and London: Routledge and Kegan Paul.

Gordon, D. (2008). *L'éveil spirituel par le rêve: guide pratique de guérison des blessures émotionnelles par le voyage mythique de transformation.* Varennes: Ada.

Gratton, N. & Séguin, M. (2011). *Dreams and Death. The benefits of dreams before, during and after death.* eBook, Montréal.

Hadfield, J. A. (1977). *Dreams and nightmares.* New York: Penguin.

Hall, J. A. (1983). *Jungian Dream Interpretation.* Toronto: Inner City books.

Hamel, J. (2001). La psychothérapie par l'art: La transformation intérieure par la voie de l'imaginaire. *Revue québécoise de psychologie, 22,* 33–48.

Hamel, J. (2017/1993). *De l'autre côté du miroir. Journal de croissance personnelle par le rêve et l'art.* Montréal: Québec-Livres.

Hamel, J. & Labrèche, J. (2015). *Art-thérapie, mettre des mots sur les maux et des couleurs sur les douleurs. La référence pour comprendre et pratiquer.* Paris: Larousse.

Hampden-Turner, C. (1982). *Maps of the mind.* New York: Collier Books/ Macmillan.

Hass-Cohen, N. & Clyde Findlay, J. (2015). *Art therapy & the Neuroscience of Relationships, Creativity and Resiliency.* New York and London: W.W. Norton.

Hennevin, E. (2003). Le rêve vu par les neurosciences. *Champ psychosomatique, 69–79.* DOI: 10.3917/cpsy.031.0069.

Hill, C. E. (1996). *Working with dreams in psychotherapy.* New York: Guilford Press.

Hill, C. E. (2010). *Working with dreams in therapy. Facilitating exploration, insight and action* (3rd ed.). Washington: American Psychological Association.

Hillman, J. (1979). *The dream and the underworld.* New York: Harper and Row.

Hillman, J. & McLean M. (1997). *Dream animals.* San Francisco: Chronicle Books.

Hobson, J. A. (1988). *The dreaming brain.* New York: Basic Book.

Hoss, R. & Gongloff, R. (Ed.) (2017). *Dreams that change our lives. A publication of the International Association for the Study of Dreams.* Asheville, NC: Chiron Publications.

International Association for the Study of Dreams (IASD). *Dreaming. Journal of the Association for the Study of Dreams.* Washington, DC: Educational Publishing Foundation.

Jacobi, Y. (1983). *The way of individuation.* New York and Ontario: Meridian.

Jobin, A.-M. (2002). *Le journal créatif.* Montréal: du Roseau.

Jobin, A.-M. (2008). *Fantaisies et gribouillis. 85 activités créatives pour tous.* Montréal: du Roseau.

Jobin, A.-M. (2010). *Le nouveau journal créatif.* Montréal: du Roseau.

Jobin, A.-M. (2013). *Créez la vie qui vous ressemble.* Montréal: Le Jour.

Johnson, R. A. (2009/1986). *Inner work. Using dreams and active imagination for personal growth.* Harper Collins ebooks.

Jung, C. G. (1989). *Memories, Dreams, Reflections.* New York: Vintage.

Jung, C. G. (1972). *Mandala symbolism.* Princeton, NJ: Bollingen Series.

Jung, C. G. (2010). *Dreams.* Princeton, NJ: Princeton University Press. Rev. Edition.

Jung, C. G. (1993). *La guérison psychologique* (6th ed.). Genève: Georg.

Jung, C. G., Shamdasani, S. et al. (2010). *The undiscovered self: With symbols and the interpretation of dreams.* Princeton: Princeton University Press.

Jung, C. G. (2012). *Man and his symbols.* Kindle Edition.

Kabat-Zinn, J. (2009). *Full catastrophe living. Using the wisdom of your body and mind to face stress, pain and illness.* New York: Bantam Dell.

Kaplan-Williams, S. (1987). *The Jungian-Senoi Dreamwork Manual: Step-By-Step Introduction to Working with Dreams.* (13e éd.). Berkeley: Journey Press.

Kelzer, K. (1990). *The sun and the shadow. My experience with lucid dreaming.* Virginia: A.R.E. Press.

Kelzer, K. (1999). *Deep journeys: Experiential psychotherapy with dreams, personal archetypal tales, and trance states.* Berkeley, CA: North Atlantic Books.

Krakow, B., Kellner, R., Pathak, D. & Lambert, L. (1996). Long term reductions in nightmares treated with imagery rehearsal. *Behavioral and cognitive psychotherapy,* 24, 135–148.

Krakow, B., Sandoval, D., Schrader, R., Keuhne, B., McBride, L., Yau, C. L. & Tandberg, D. (2001). Treatment of chronic nightmares in adjudicated adolescent girls in a residential facility. *Journal of Adolescent Health* 29(2), 94–100.

Krakow, B. & Zadra, A. (2004). Clinical management of chronic nightmares: Imagery rehearsal therapy. *Behavioral sleep medicine,* 1, 45–70.

Krippner, S. (Ed.). (1991). *Dreamtime and dreamwork. Decoding the language of the night.* Los Angeles: Tarcher.

Laberge, S. & Rheingold, H. (1990). *Exploring the world of lucid dreaming.* New York: Ballantine Books.

Laberge, S. (1999). *Le rêve lucide. Le pouvoir de l'éveil et de la conscience dans vos rêves.* Centre de recherche sur le sommeil de l'université Stanford: Oniros.

Laberge, S. (1985). *Lucid Dreaming. The power of being awake and aware in your dreams.* New York: Balllantine Books.

Laberge, S. (2008). *S'éveiller en rêvant. Introduction au rêve lucide.* Paris: Almora.

Lévesque, A.-M. (2015). L'approche jungienne en art-thérapie. In: Hamel, J. & Labrèche, J. (eds) *Art-thérapie, mettre des mots sur les maux et des couleurs sur les douleurs. La référence pour comprendre et pratiquer.* Paris: Larousse.

Magallòn, L. L. & Shor, B. (1991). Shared dreaming: Joining together in dreamtime. In: Krippner, S. (ed.) *Dreamtime and dreamwork, Decoding the language of the night.* Los Angeles: Tarcher.

Martin, S. A. (1992). Smaller Than Small, Bigger than Big: The Role of the 'Little Dream' in Individuation. *Quadrant* XXV: 2.

Mattoon, M. A. (1978). *Applied Dream Analysis. A Jungian Approach.* Washington: V. H. Winston and Sons.

Mattoon, M. A. (1984). *Understanding dreams.* Dallas: Spring Publications.

McMurray, M. (1988). *Illumination. The healing image.* California: Wingbow.

Mellick, J. (1996). *The natural artistry of dreams: Creative ways to bring the wisdom of dream to waking life.* Berkeley: Conari Press.

Mellick, J. (2001/1996). *The art of dreaming: Tools for creative dream work.* Berkeley: Conari Press.

Mindell, A. (1982). *Dreambody. The body's role in revealing the Self.* Santa Monica: Sigo Press.

Mindell, A. (1985). *Working with the dreaming body.* Boston: Routledge and Kegan Paul.

Morley, C. (2013). *Dreams of awakening: Lucid dreaming and mindfulness of dream and sleep.* London: Hay House.

Morris, J. (2002/1985). *The Dream workbook.* Boston: Little, Brown and Company

Neu, E. R. (1988). *Dreams and dream groups. Messages from the interior.* California: Crossing Press/Freedom.

Ochs, L. V. & Ochs, E. (2003). *The Jewish dream book. The key to opening the inner meaning of your dreams.* Woodstock: Jewish Lights Publishing.

Pearce, J. C. (2002). *The crack in the cosmic egg.* Toronto: Simon and Schuster Canada.

Perls, F. (1970). «*Four lectures*» in Gestalt therapy now. Theory, techniques, applications. Palo Alto: Science and Behavior.

Perls, F. (1972). *In and out of the garbage pail.* New York: Bantam Books. 2nd printing.

Perls, F. (1992/1969). *Gestalt Therapy Verbatim.* Highland, NY: Gestalt Journal.

Pesant, N. & Zadra, A. (2004). Working with dreams in therapy: What do we know and what should we do? *Clinical Psychology Review*, 24, 489–512.

Pesant, N. & Zadra, A. (2006). Évaluation de l'utilité clinique de séances d'interprétation du rêve basées sur un modèle cognitif-expérientiel. *Revue québécoise de psychologie*, 27(1), 153–170.

Pesant, N. & Zadra, A. (2010). L'utilisation des rêves en psychothérapie: Une approche intégrative. *Revue québécoise de psychologie*, 31(2), 9–31.

Petschek, J. (1981). *The silver bird. A tale for those who dream.* Berkeley, CA: Celestial Arts.

Polster, I. & M. (1983). *La gestalt, nouvelles perspectives théoriques et choix thérapeutiques et éducatifs.* Montréal: Le jour.

Polster, I. & Polster, M. (1974). *Gestalt therapy integrated.* New York: Vintage Books.

Reed, H. (1985). *Getting help from your dreams.* New York: Ballantine Books.

Rhyne, J. (1984). *The gestalt art experience.* California: Magnolia Street.

Rhinehart, L. & Engelhorn, F. (1982). *Class notes on sandtray. Art therapy training*. Santa Rosa: Eagle Rock Trail Art Therapy Institute.

Rhinehart, L. & Engelhorn, F. (1987). *Sandtray dialogue*. Santa Rosa: Rainbow Bridges.

Rhinehart, L. & Engelhorn, F. (1992). Pre-image considerations as a therapeutic process. *The Arts in Psychotherapy, 9*, 55–63.

Rinfret, M. (1992). *Caractéristiques du travail sur le rêve à partir des sons et des mouvements*. Sherbrooke: Texte inédit.

Rogers, C. (1961). *On becoming a person: A therapist's view of psychotherapy*. Boston: Houghton Mifflin Harcourt.

Rohnnberg, A. & Martin, K. (2011). (Ed.) *Le livre des symboles. Réflexions sur des images archétypales*. Köln: Taschen.

Romey, G. (2005). *Dictionnaire de la symbolique des rêves*. Paris: Albin Michel.

Rossi, E. L. (2000). *Dreams consciousness spirit. The Quantum experience of self-reflection and co-creation*. Malibu, CA: Palisades Gateway Publishing.

Sams, J. & Carson, D. (1988). *Medicine Cards*. Santa Fe, New Mexico: Bear and Company.

Schwartz-Salant, N. and Murray, S. (1990). *Dreams in analysis*. Wilmette, IL: Chiron.

Shafton, A. (1995). *Dream reader: contemporary approaches to the understanding of dreams*. Albany, NY: State University of New York Press.

Shainberg, C. (2005). *Kabbalah and the power of dreaming. Awakening the visionary life*. Rochester, VT: Inner Traditions.

Sher, E. (1978). *A child's library of dreams*. Berkeley: Celestial Arts.

Signell, K. A. (1990). *Wisdom of the heart. Working with women's dreams*. New York: Bantam.

Simard, V. & Nielsen, T. A. (2009). Adaptation of imagery rehearsal therapy for nightmares in children: A brief report. *Psychotherapy: Theory, Research, Practice, Training, 46*(4), 492–497.

Sparrow, G. S. (1992/1982). *Lucid dreaming. Dawning of the clear light* (2nd ed.). Virginia: A.R.E.

Stein, M. (2009). Symbol as Psychic Transformer. *Symbolic Life, a Journal of Archetype and Culture, 82*, 1–11.

Sun Bear. (1983). *The Path of Power*. Washington: Bear Tribe.

Tart, C. T. (1986). *Waking up, Overcoming the Obstacles to Human Potential*. Boston: New Science Library.

Taylor, J. (2009). *The Wisdom of Your Dreams. Using Dreams to Tap into Your Unconscious and Transform Your Life*. New York: Penguin.

Taylor, J. (1992). *Where people fly and water runs uphill. Using dreams to tap the wisdom of the unconscious*. New York: Warner.

Taylor, J. (1983). *Dream work. Techniques for discovering the creative power in dreams*. New York/Ramsey: Paulist Press.

Tolaas, J. (1991). The Puzzle of Psychic Dreaming. In: Krippner, S. (ed.) *Dreamtime and dreamwork, decoding the language of the night*. Los Angeles: Tarcher.

Turner, B. A. (2005). *The Handbook Of Sandplay Therapy*. Cloverdale: Temenos Press.

Ullman, M. & Zimmerman, N. (1979). *Working With Dreams: Self-Understanding, Problem-Solving And Enriched Creativity Through Dream Appreciation*. Los Angeles: Jeremy P. Tarcher.

Vaughan-Lee, L. (1990). *The lover and the serpent. Dreamwork within a sufi tradition*. Longmead, Dorset, England: Element.

Viens, S. (2015). L'art-thérapie et le travail des rêves. In: Hamel, J. & Labrèche, J. (eds). *Art-thérapie, mettre des mots sur les maux et des couleurs sur les douleurs. La référence pour comprendre et pratiquer*. Paris: Larousse.

Von Franz, M.-L. (1983). *Alchemical Active Imagination*. Zurich: Spring.

Von Franz, M.-L. (1992). *Rêves d'hier et d'aujourd'hui*. Paris: Albin Michel.

Von Franz, M.-L. (2008). *La voie des rêves*. Ville d'Avray: La fontaine de Pierre.

Waggoner, R. & McCready, C. (2015). *Lucid Dreaming, Plain and Simple. Tips and Techniques for Insight, Creativity and Personal Growth*. San Francisco: Conary.

Waggoner, R. (1973). *Lucid Dreaming. Gateway to the Inner Self*. Needham, MA: Moment Point.

Watkins, M. (1984). *Waking Dreams*. Zurich: Spring Publications.

Weinrib, E. (2004). *Images of the Self: The Sandtray Therapy Process*. Hot Springs, AR: Temenos Press.

Wilkinson, M. (2006). The Dreaming Mind-Brain: A Jungian Perspective. *Journal of Analytical Psychology*, 51, 43–59.

Windsor, J. (1987). *Dreams Healing*. New York: Dodd, Mead and Company.

Wolf, F. A. (1994). *The Dreaming Universe*. New York: Simon and Schuster.

Woodman, M. (1991). *Dreams: Language of the Soul*. [Audio]. Boulder, CO: Sounds True Recordings.

Zadra, A. & Pihl, R. O. (1997). Lucid Dreaming: A Treatment For Recurrent Nightmares. *Psychotherapy and Psychosomatics*, 65(1), 50–55.

Zwig, A. (1991). A Body-Oriented Approach To Dreamwork. In: Krippner, S. (Ed.). *Dreamtime and dreamwork. Decoding the language of the night*. Los Angeles: Tarcher, 78–92.

Author's Index

Words and Expressions' Index